Living Well with
HIV & AIDS

Allen L. Gifford, M.D.

Kate Lorig, R.N., Dr. P.H.

Diana Laurent, M.P.H.

Virginia Gonzaléz, M.P.H.

Bull Publishing Company
Palo Alto, CA

Copyright ©1997 Bull Publishing Company

Bull Publishing Company
P.O. Box 208
Palo Alto, CA 94302-0208
Phone (415) 322-2855   Fax (415) 327-3300

ISBN 0-923521-35-6

Distributed to the trade by:
Publishers Group West
4065 Hollis Street
Emeryville, CA 94608

Publisher: James Bull
Production Manager: Helen O'Donnell
Production: Mary Douglas, Rogue Valley Publications
Cover Design: Robb Pawlak, Pawlak Design
Interior Design: Linda Robertson
Composition: Susan Benoit & Associates

Library of Congress Cataloging-in-Publication Data

Living well with HIV & AIDS / Allen L. Gifford . . . [et al.].
    p. cm.
  Includes bibliographical references and index.
  ISBN 0-923521-35-6 (alk. paper)
  1. AIDS (Disease)—Popular works. 2. Self-care. Health.
I. Gifford, Allen L.
RC607.A26.L587 1996   96-13730
362.1′969792—dc20

Brief Contents

Detailed Contents

Acknowledgments

This book was produced with the help of many people. First and foremost for acknowledgment are the efforts of the many people with HIV/AIDS, and their friends and families, who have made suggestions about things that should be included in this book and ways to improve it. And many of the ideas included here are from doctors, nurses, health educators, and other health professionals who have devoted themselves to improving the lives of people with HIV/AIDS.

None of the work represented here would be possible without the support of the Lawrence S. Linn Research Trust, the Clinical Scholar Program of the Robert Wood Johnson Foundation, and the Department of Veterans Affairs.

Certain individuals require special mention. Chris Adams helped conceive and plan this project, and his intelligence, wit, and bravery in facing his own illness inspired us all. Special thanks also go to Peg Harrison, Halsted Holman, Marian Minor, David Sobel, and all the extraordinary nurses, staff, and physicians of the Infectious Disease Specialty Practice of the University of California, San Francisco.

to Chris Adams

How to Use This Book

No one wants to have HIV or AIDS. But just because you have HIV/AIDS* doesn't mean that life comes to an end. This book has been written to help people with HIV/AIDS learn a healthy way to live. Now this may seem like a strange concept. How can one have an illness and live a healthy life at the same time? To answer this question, it is important to think about what "health" really is: *Health is soundness of body and mind, and a healthy life is a life which seeks that soundness.* Therefore, a healthy way to live with any illness is to work at overcoming the physical and emotional problems caused by the illness. The goal is to achieve the greatest possible physical capability and pleasure from life. People with all kinds of illnesses do this successfully every day. That is what this book is all about.

But can people with HIV/AIDS live healthy lives? Of course. HIV/AIDS is a chronic disease like many others. It has many similarities with conditions like diabetes and heart disease, just to name two. If HIV/AIDS becomes symptomatic, it causes decreased function of the immune system. The chronic symptoms that may result can cause people to lose physical conditioning. In addition, these symptoms may cause feelings of emotional distress, such as depression, frustration, or helplessness. All these things can affect how life is lived. The job of the person living with HIV/AIDS is to find ways to deal with these symptoms and decrease the effects of HIV on life. To do this well, you need to be involved in planning and decision making about how you're going to live with your illness. You need to be a *self-manager.*

You will not find any miracles or cures in these pages. Rather, you will

---

*The terminology used in discussing HIV-related disease is clumsy. We don't want to just use the term *AIDS* because this would exclude people with earlier HIV infection and ARC (AIDS-related complex). Therefore, throughout this book, we will often use the term *HIV/AIDS* to refer in general to the full range of conditions caused by HIV infection.

find tips, ideas, and resources about how to become an HIV/AIDS self-manager and make your life better. This advice comes from physicians, health professionals, psychologists, and, most importantly, from people like you who have learned to manage living with their HIV/AIDS. Part 1 of the book (HIV/AIDS Self-Management) will introduce you to the concepts and skills you need to become an HIV/AIDS self-manager. Part 2 (Managing Symptoms) will help you evaluate and begin to control some of the symptoms you may experience. Part 3 (Managing Exercise and Diet) contains information about a healthy approach to exercising and eating. Part 4 (Managing Health Care) will help you manage the health care system better. And Part 5 (Managing Practical Details) will help you better handle the tasks of daily life that can become so complicated when you're living with a chronic condition.

HIV/AIDS affects the lives of all kinds of people, with differing personal histories, sexual preferences, and cultural backgrounds. Also, HIV/AIDS affects people if they're HIV-positive without symptoms as well as if they develop symptoms or AIDS illnesses. And the people that *care about* people with HIV/AIDS and live with them and care for them—these people are also affected. This book will be helpful for all these people.

This is not a "textbook"—you don't have to sit down and read every word in every chapter. Instead, read the next two chapters and then use the table of contents to find what you need. Many people pick and choose; feel free to skip around. You may want to start with some background information from the third part of the book about HIV/AIDS and its symptoms and treatments. People who don't have symptoms may want to start by learning about exercise, healthy eating, and stress reduction. And people with all stages of HIV can use the knowledge here to help figure out whether a new symptom is a regular "bug" or an urgent condition that needs to be checked out by the doctor. Become familiar with the information in the different sections, and use it in the order that's helpful for you.

The resources available for people with HIV/AIDS are always changing, so while we hope that the "leads" given here will be useful, they may just be good starting points. If you have any good tips or helpful hints you want to pass on to others, please write us at the address below. We will incorporate them into future editions of this book.

Please send your ideas or tips to:

The Stanford Patient Education Research Center
1000 Welch Road, Suite 204
Palo Alto, CA 94304

E-mail: DDL@dbn.stanford.edu

HIV/AIDS
Self-Management

1

Overview of HIV/AIDS Self-Management

HIV/AIDS is a chronic disease like many others. But what does this mean? To learn to be an HIV/AIDS self-manager, it's important to know how acute and chronic diseases differ and why those differences are important.

Acute and Chronic Conditions

We think of a health problem as being either "acute" or "chronic." Acute health problems usually begin abruptly with a single, easily diagnosed cause; they last for a limited time, and they respond to a specific treatment, such as medication or surgery. For most acute illnesses, a cure with return to normal health is to be expected. For the patient and the doctor, there is relatively little uncertainty. One usually knows what to expect. The illness typically has a cycle of getting worse for a while, being treated, and then getting better. The care of an acute illness depends on a health professional's knowledge and experience to find and administer the correct treatment.

Appendicitis is an example of an acute illness, which typically begins rapidly, signaled by nausea and pain in the abdomen. The diagnosis of appendicitis, established by physical examination, leads to surgery for removal of the inflamed appendix. There follows a period of recovery and then a return to normal health.

Chronic illnesses are different. They begin slowly and proceed slowly. For example, a person with arteriosclerosis ("hardening of the arteries") might have chest pains or breathing problems. Most arthritis starts with little annoying twinges, which gradually increase. Unlike acute disease, chronic illnesses have multiple causes varying over time and include heredity, lifestyle factors (smoking, lack of exercise, poor diet, stress, and so on), exposure to environmental factors, and physiological factors.

HIV/AIDS is a chronic disease and in many ways is quite similar to other chronic diseases, such as heart disease, stroke, or diabetes. But HIV/AIDS is a chronic illness that is sometimes interrupted by acute infections or conditions. For example, a person with HIV may have day-in, day-out chronic symptoms of fatigue and then may have a brief, acute episode of *Pneumocystis* pneumonia. Knowing the difference between the acute conditions and the chronic conditions associated with HIV/AIDS is quite important, because the acute conditions are sometimes infections ("opportunistic" infections) that need special treatment.

Chronic symptoms with multiple causes can be frustrating for those of us who want quick answers. It is difficult for the doctor and the patient when immediate answers aren't available. In some cases, even when diagnosis is rapid, such as in the case of a stroke or heart attack, long-term effects may be hard to predict. The lack of a regular or predictable pattern is a major characteristic in most chronic illness, and especially in HIV/AIDS.

Unlike acute disease, in which full recovery is expected, chronic illness usually leads to persistent loss of physical conditioning. Because chronically ill people tire easily, they are unable to accomplish what they once could. They are forced to give up recreational activities, such as walking or going to the gym, or chores like shopping, housework, and yard work. This lack of activity accelerates physical deconditioning. At the same time, the loss of

Acute Versus Chronic Conditions		
Example	*Acute Conditions* *Pneumocystis* Pneumonia	*Chronic Conditions* Fatigue
Beginning	Rapid	Gradual
Duration	Short	Indefinite
Treatment	Cure common	Cure rare
Role of professional	Select and conduct therapy	Teach and advise
Role of patient	Follow professional's instructions/advice	Active partner of health professionals, responsible for daily management

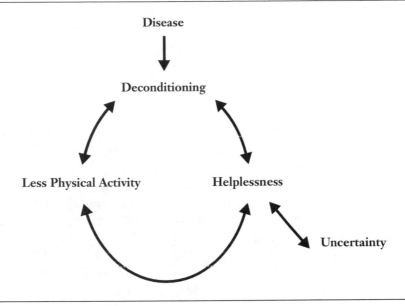

Figure 1.1   The Cycle of Deconditioning

physical activity and uncertainty about the future create a sense of helplessness, a feeling that little or nothing can be done to help the situation. Of course, believing nothing can be done is a guarantee that nothing will be done, reinforcing helplessness and perpetuating the vicious cycle. A primary problem of living with HIV/AIDS is dealing with this cycle of physical deconditioning and helplessness. Throughout this book we examine ways of breaking the cycle and stopping the physical deconditioning and helplessness that have been started by chronic illness.

What Causes a Chronic Disease?

To answer this question, we need to understand how the body operates. As you know, cells are the building blocks of tissues and organs: the heart, lungs, brain, blood, blood vessels, bones, muscles—in fact, everything in the body. For a cell to remain alive and function normally, three things must happen: it must be nourished, receive oxygen, and get rid of waste products. If anything goes wrong with any of these three functions, the cell is diseased. When cells are diseased, the organ or tissue suffers, which may lead to limitations in your ability to be active in daily life. The difference in chronic diseases depends on which cells and organs are affected and the processes by which the effect occurs. For example, in a stroke, a blood vessel in the brain becomes blocked or breaks. Oxygen and nutrition are cut off from part of the brain, and as a result, the parts of your body controlled by the damaged brain cells, such as an arm or a leg or a portion of the face, lose function.

If you have heart disease, several things might happen. For instance, heart attacks occur when the blood vessels supplying blood to the heart muscle become blocked. This is called a coronary thrombosis (*thrombos* means "clot"). When this happens, oxygen is cut off, the heart muscle is injured, and pain results. After the injury, the heart may be less effective in supplying the rest of your body with oxygen-carrying blood. Because the heart is pumping blood less efficiently through the body, fluid accumulates in tissues, and shortness of breath occurs.

With bronchitis, asthma, and emphysema, there is either a problem getting oxygen to the lungs, as with bronchitis or asthma, or the lungs cannot effectively transfer oxygen to the blood, as in emphysema. In both cases the body is deprived of oxygen.

Chronic HIV/AIDS can be similar to these diseases in the sense that damage to the immune system may lead to problems with the lungs and the body may be deprived of oxygen. The basic consequences of stroke, heart disease, and lung disease are similar: loss of function due to a reduction in oxygen. But HIV can also lead to loss of function in other ways. Nerve cell damage caused by the virus can cause numbness or discomfort in the feet and hands. Problems in the intestines may decrease the absorption of fluids and important nutrients. Furthermore, the overall work that the body has to do to fight HIV in the cells can lead to an energy drain and fatigue. These things don't always happen, but if any one of them does, it can lead to pain and disability.

Although all chronic illness starts at a cellular level, one does not always know that a disease is present until the symptoms start (shortness of breath, fatigue, pain, and so on). Illness is more than cellular malfunction. It also includes the problems of everyday life, such as not being able to do the things you want to do or needing to change your social activities.

Though the biological causes of chronic diseases differ, the problems they cause for patients are similar. For example, most people with chronic disease suffer fatigue and loss of energy. Sleeping problems are not uncommon. Some people may have pain, whereas others may have trouble breathing. Disability, to some extent, is a part of chronic disease. It may be an inability to use your hands well because of arthritis or stroke, or difficulty in walking due to shortness of breath, stroke, or arthritis.

Another common problem with chronic illness is depression, or just "feeling blue." It is hard to have a cheerful disposition when your condition causes problems that probably won't go away. Along with the depression come fear and concern for the future. Will I be able to remain independent? If I can't care for myself, who will care for me? What will happen to my family? Will I get worse? Disability and depression bring loss of self-esteem.

Finally, because of similarities among chronic illnesses, the central management tasks and skills one must learn to live with all chronic illness are similar. Besides overcoming the physical and emotional problems, it is important to learn problem-solving skills and how to respond to the trends in your disease. These tasks and skills include developing and maintaining health with appropriate exercise and nutrition, managing symptoms, making decisions about when to seek medical help, working effectively with your doctor, using medications and minimizing side effects, finding and using community resources, talking about your illness with family and friends, and if necessary, changing social interactions. The most important skill of all is learning to respond to your illness on an ongoing basis to solve day-to-day problems as they arise.

Chronic illnesses, including HIV/AIDS, have more in common than first meets the eye. In this book, we talk about managing HIV/AIDS as well as how to use the principles that have been successful in managing other chronic illnesses. Before we discuss management techniques, however, it is necessary to explain what we mean by self-management.

The Path of Chronic Illness

The first responsibility of any manager is to understand what is being managed. Initially, this may seem like an impossible task. After all, HIV/AIDS is a very complicated and challenging disease that sometimes stumps the best of specialists. But understanding HIV/AIDS is not as difficult as it might seem to the newcomer, for two reasons. First, as a result of daily living with the consequences of the illness, you and your family will become familiar with the effects of the disease and the treatments, and with the ways the treatments are used. With experience, you may become better than health professionals at judging your disease and treatment consequences. Second, most chronic illnesses go up and down in intensity; they do not have a steady path. Therefore, being able to identify the ups and downs in the path accurately is essential for good management.

For example, the letters *A*, *B*, and *C* in Figure 1.2 represent a particular

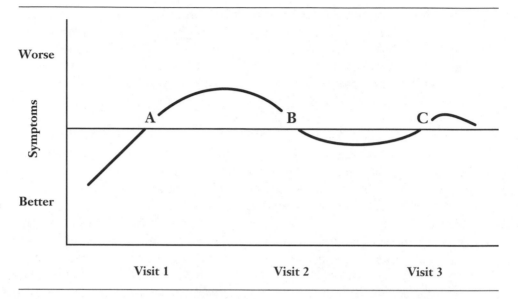

Figure 1.2   The Path of Chronic Illness

symptom. As you can see, even though all three letters are at the same level of intensity at each visit, they can mean entirely different things when your health care team is evaluating whether to maintain or change treatment. In the case of *A*, the disease is worsening, so additional treatment may be in order. In the case of *B*, things seem to be getting better, so keeping the treatment stable or even lessening it may be the choice. In the case of *C*, things have been stable for a while, so maintaining treatment may be the best treatment option.

Your experience and understanding communicated clearly to the physician are often the best indicators of the path's course, and skilled clinicians commonly depend upon them. Frequently, your experience of how you are doing is a better indicator than laboratory tests or other measures. If the clinician encourages and facilitates your learning and you respond by participating in decisions, a partnership is born. To be most effective, self-management in HIV/AIDS requires such a partnership.

When you develop any chronic illness, you become more aware of your body. Minor symptoms that were formerly ignored may now cause great concern. For example, is this cough a signal of a pneumonia? Is this pain in my leg a sign that neuropathy (chronic nerve pain) has started? There are no simple, reassuring answers to apply to all patients. Nor is there a failsafe way of sorting out serious signals from minor temporary symptoms that can be ignored. It is helpful to understand the natural rhythms of your chronic illness. In general, symptoms should be checked out with your doctor if they are *unusual, severe, persistent,* or *occur after starting a new medication.* Some other guidelines are provided in Chapter 3, "Evaluating Common Symptoms of HIV."

Throughout this book, we give some specific examples of what actions to take if you experience certain symptoms. But this is where your partnership with your doctor becomes most critical. He or she can help guide you in responding to specific problems or symptoms. Self-management does not mean going it alone. Get help or advice when you are concerned or uncertain.

The Job of Self-Management

In terms of what has just been said, self-management may seem like a simple-enough term. Both at home and in the business world, managers direct the show. They don't do everything themselves; they work with others, including consultants, to get the job done. What makes them managers is that *they are responsible* for making the decisions and making sure these decisions are carried out. As a manager of your illness, your job is much the same. You gather information and hire a consultant or a team of consultants consisting of your physician, other health professionals, and support people such as family and friends. Once they have given you their best advice, it is up to you to follow through. All chronic illness needs day-to-day management. We have all noticed that some people with severe physical problems get on well, whereas others with lesser problems seem to give up on life. The difference is often attitude and management style.

Managing a chronic illness, like managing a family or a business, is a complex undertaking. There are many twists, turns, and midcourse corrections. By learning self-management skills, you can ease the problems of living with your condition.

The keys to success in any undertaking are:

- deciding what you want to do
- deciding how you are going to do it
- learning a set of skills and practicing until you have mastered them

These tasks are all based on your learning skills and mastering them. Success in HIV/AIDS self-management is the same. In fact, mastering such skills is one of the most important tasks of life.

We will describe several skills and strategies to help relieve the problems caused by HIV/AIDS. We do not expect you to use all of them. Pick and choose. Experiment. Set your own goals. What you do may not be as important as the sense of confidence and control that comes from successfully doing something you want to do. However, we have learned that knowing the skills is not enough. You need a way of incorporating these skills into your daily life. Whenever we try a new skill, the first attempts are usually clumsy and slow and show few results. It is easier to return to old ways than to continue trying to master new and sometimes difficult tasks. The best way to master new skills is through practice and evaluation of the results.

Self-Management Skills

What you do about something is largely determined by how you think about it. For example, some people think that having HIV is like having a heavy weight hanging overhead that won't ever go away and that might fall at any time. Thinking like that, such people might never try to control what happens to them. They might even think it's useless to do anything at all. The thoughts you have can greatly determine what happens to you and how you handle your health problems.

Some of the most successful self-managers are people who think of their illness as a path. This path, like any path, goes up and down. Sometimes it is flat and smooth. At other times the way is rough. To negotiate this path you have to use many strategies. Sometimes you can go fast; other times you must slow down. There are obstacles to negotiate. Good self-managers are people who have learned the skills to negotiate this path.

Self-management skills fall into three main categories:

- *Skills needed to deal with the illness.* Any illness requires that you do new things. These may include taking medicine, using an inhaler, or using oxygen. Illness means more frequent interactions with your doctor and the health care system. Sometimes there are new exercises or a new diet. All of these constitute the work you must do to manage your illness.

- *Skills needed to continue your normal life.* Just because you have HIV does not mean that life stops. There are still chores to do, friendships to maintain, jobs to go to, and a multitude of family relationships to carry on. Things that you once took for granted can become much more complicated in the face of HIV/AIDS. You may need to learn new skills in order to maintain your daily activities and to enjoy life.

- *Skills needed to deal with emotions.* When you are diagnosed as having HIV/AIDS, your future changes, and with this come changes in plans and changes in emotions. Many of these emotions are negative. They may include anger ("Why me? It's not fair"); depression ("I can't do anything anymore. What's the use?"); frustration ("No matter what I do, it doesn't make any difference. I can't do what I want to do"); or isolation ("No one understands. No one wants to be around someone who is sick"). Negotiating the path of HIV, then, also means learning skills to work with these negative emotions.

Self-Management Tasks

- *Taking care of your illness* (Taking medicine, exercising, going to the doctor, changing diet)

- *Carrying out your normal activities* (Household chores, employment, social life, and so on)

- *Managing your emotional changes* (Changes brought about by your illness, such as anger, uncertainty about the future, changed expectations and goals, and sometimes depression. Changes can also happen in your relationship with family and friends.)

2

Becoming an HIV/AIDS Self-Manager

Like any skill, self-management must be learned and practiced. This chapter will start you on your way. Remember, *you are the manager.* Like the manager of an organization or household, you must have a management plan:

1. *Decide* what you want to accomplish.
2. *Look for alternative ways* to accomplish this goal.
3. Start making short-term plans by *making a contract* or agreement with yourself.
4. *Carry out your contract.*
5. *Check the results.*
6. *Make changes* as needed.
7. Remember to *reward yourself.*

Problems sometimes start with a general uneasiness. You are unhappy but not sure why. Upon closer examination, you find you miss contact with some distant relatives. With the problem identified, you decide to take a trip to visit your relatives. You know what you *want to accomplish.* In the past, you have always driven, but now find it tiring, so you seek *alternative ways* of travel. Among other things, you consider leaving at noon instead of early in the morning and making the trip in two days instead of one. You consider asking a friend along to share the driving. There is also a train that goes within twenty miles of your destination, or you might fly (although the airport is not very convenient). You decide to take the train. The trip still seems overwhelming, as there is so much to do to prepare. You decide to write down all the steps necessary to make the trip a reality. These include finding a good time to go, buying a ticket, figuring out how to handle luggage, seeing if you can make it up and down the stairs to get on the train, considering whether you can walk on a moving train to get food or to the bathroom, and thinking about how you can manage your medications when you're away from home.

You start by *making a contract* or agreement with yourself that this week you will call and find out just how much the railroad can help. You also decide to start taking a short walk each day and to walk up and down a few steps so you can be steadier on your feet. You then *carry out your contract* by calling the railroad and starting your walking program.

A week later, you *check the results.* Looking back at all the steps to be accomplished, you find that a single call answered many questions. The railroad is used to people who have mobility problems and has dealt with many of your concerns. However, you are still worried about walking. Even though you are walking better, you are still unsteady. You *make a change in your plan* by asking a physical therapist about this, and he suggests using a cane. Although you hate to do it, you find that a cane gives you that extra security needed on a moving train. As a reward to yourself for your efforts, you buy an attractive wooden cane to replace the metal one from physical therapy.

Now you are ready to make a new contract for accomplishing some of the other tasks necessary to make the trip possible. What once seemed like a dream has become a reality.

Now let's go through these seven steps in detail. They are the backbone of any self-management program.

Deciding What You Want to Accomplish

Deciding what you want to accomplish may be the most difficult part. You must be realistic and very specific. Think of all the things you would like to do. One of our self-managers wanted to climb twenty steps to his friend's home so he could join his friend's family for a holiday meal. Another wanted to gain weight to improve his strength. Still another wanted to be more socially active but felt limited by the need to take an oxygen tank everywhere. In each case, the goal was one that would take several weeks or even months to accomplish. In fact, one of the problems with goals is that they often seem like dreams. They are so far off that we don't even try to accomplish them. We'll tackle this problem next. For now, take a moment to write your goals below. When you have finished, put an asterisk (*) next to the goal you would like to work on first.

Goals

1. _____
2. _____
3. _____

Looking for Alternative Ways of Accomplishing the Goal

Sometimes what keeps us from reaching our goal is a failure to see alternatives. Other times, we reject alternatives without knowing much about them.

There are many ways to reach any specific goal. For example, our self-manager who wanted to climb twenty steps could start off with a slow walking program, start to climb a few steps each day, or look into having the family gathering at a different place. The man who wanted to gain weight could decide to keep a log of his daily calorie intake, talk to his doctor about changing some of his medications, or start an exercise program. The self-manager who wanted more social contact could find out about community college classes, support groups, or could call or write friends.

As you can see, there are many options for reaching each goal. The job here is to list the options and then choose one or two on which you would like to work. Sometimes it is hard to think of all the options yourself. If you are having problems, it is time to use a consultant. Share your goal with family, friends, and health professionals. You can call community organizations such as your local AIDS Foundation or Project Inform.* But rather than asking *what* you should do, ask for *suggestions*. It is always good to have a list of options.

Many options are never seriously considered because you assume they don't exist or are not workable. Try not to make this assumption until you have thoroughly investigated the option. One woman we know had lived in the same town all her life and felt that she knew all about the community resources. When she was having problems with her health insurance, a friend from another city suggested contacting an insurance counselor. The woman dismissed this suggestion, however, because she *knew* that this service did not exist in her town. Months later the friend came to visit and called the area

---

*These are just two out of many community and national organizations available to people with HIV/AIDS and their friends and families. There's more information about these resources in Chapter 16.

social service agencies (listed in the telephone book) and located three insurance counseling services. In short, never assume anything. Assumptions are the major enemies to the self-manager.

Once you have identified your options, write them below and put an asterisk (*) next to the two or three options on which you would like to work first.

Options

1. _____
2. _____
3. _____
4. _____
5. _____
6. _____

Making Short-Term Plans—Contracting

The next step is to turn your options into *short-term plans*, which we will call a *contract*. A contract calls for a specific action or set of actions that you can realistically expect to accomplish within the next week. The contract should be about something *you* want to do or accomplish. This is a tool to help you do what *you* wish. You do not make contracts to please your friends, family, or doctor, but rather to please yourself. Contracts are probably your most important self-management tool. Most of us can do things to make ourselves healthier, but we fail to do them. For example, most people with chronic illness can walk—some just across the room, others for half a block. Most can walk several blocks, and some can walk a mile or more. However, few people have a systematic exercise program. A contract helps you to do the things you know you should do. Knowing how to make a realistic contract is an important skill that may well determine the success of your self-management program:

1. First, *decide what you will do* this week. For a step climber, this might be climbing three steps in four days. The man trying to gain weight may decide to eat six meals per day, each in smaller amounts than usual so that they don't upset his stomach. This action must be something *you* want to do, that you feel you can do realistically, a step on the way to your long-term goal. Make sure that your plans are *behavior-specific*—that is, rather than "relax," you will "listen to my progressive muscle relaxation tapes."

2. Next, *make a specific plan.* This is the most difficult and important part of making a contract. Deciding what you want to do is worthless without a plan to do it. The plan should contain all of the following parts:

- Exactly *what* are you going to do? How far will you walk, how will you eat less, what breathing technique will you practice?

- *How much* will you do? Will you walk around the block, walk for 15 minutes, practice breathing exercises for 15 minutes?

- *When* will you do this? Again, this must be specific: before lunch, in the shower, when I come home from work? Connecting a new activity with an old habit is a good way to make sure it gets done. Another trick is to schedule your new activity before an old favorite activity, such as reading the paper or watching a favorite TV program.

- *How often* will you do the activity? This is a bit tricky. We would all like to do things every day. However, we are human, and it is not always possible. It is usually best to contract to do something three or four times a week. If you do more, so much the better. However, if you are like most of us, you can do your activity three or four times and still be successful at your contract. **Please note!!** Taking medications is an exception. This must be done exactly as you and your doctor have agreed. Otherwise you will never know whether the medications can help, and you might put yourself in great danger.

There are a couple of guidelines for writing your contract that may help you achieve success:

- *Start where you are, or start slowly.* If you can walk only for 1 minute, start your walking program with walking 1 minute once every hour or two, not with walking a mile. If you have never done any exercise, start with a few minutes of warm-up. A total of 5 or 10 minutes is enough. If you want to lose weight, set a goal based on your eating behaviors, such as not eating after dinner.

- *Give yourself some time off.* All people have days when they don't feel like doing anything. It is better to say you will do something three times a week instead of every day. That way, if you don't feel like walking one day, you can still meet your contract.

Once you've made your contract, ask yourself the following question: "On a scale of 0 to 10, with 0 being totally unsure and 10 being totally confident, how confident am I that I can complete this contract?"

Aspects of a Contract

1. Something *you* want to do
2. Reasonable (something you can expect to be able to accomplish that week)
3. Behavior-specific
4. Answers the questions:

   What?
   How much?
   When? (Think about your day/week—which days, times?)
   How often?
5. Confidence level of 7 or more (that you will complete the *entire* contract)

If your answer is 7 or above, yours is probably a realistic contract. Congratulate yourself—you have done the hard work. If your answer is below 7, then you should look again at your contract. Ask yourself why you're not confident. What problems do you foresee? Then see if you can either solve the problems or change your contract to make yourself more confident of success.

Once you have made a contract you are happy with, write it down and post it where you will see it every day. Keep track of how you are doing and the problems you encounter. We've included an example of a contract form at the end of this chapter. You may want to make copies of it to use weekly.

Carrying Out Your Contract

If the contract is well written and realistic, fulfilling it is generally pretty easy. Ask family or friends to check with you on how you are doing. Having to report your progress is good motivation. Keep track of your daily activities while carrying out your plan. All good managers have lists of what they want to accomplish. Check things off as they are completed. This will give you guidance on how realistic your planning was and will also be useful in making future plans. Make daily notes, even of the things you don't understand at the time. Later these notes may be useful in establishing a pattern to use for problem solving.

For example, our stair-climbing friend never did his climbing. Each day he had a different problem: not enough time, being tired, the weather was too cold, and so on. When he looked back at his notes, he began to realize that the real problem was his fear of falling with no one around to help him. He then decided to use a cane while climbing stairs and to do it when a friend or neighbor was around.

Checking the Results

At the end of each week, see if you completed your contract and if you are any nearer to accomplishing your goal. Are you able to walk farther? Have you gained weight? Are you less fatigued? Taking stock is important. You may not see progress day by day, but you should see a little progress each week. At the end of each week, check on how well you have fulfilled your contract. If you are having problems, this is the time to problem-solve.

Making Midcourse Changes—Problem Solving

When you are trying to overcome obstacles, your first plan may not always be the most usable plan. If something doesn't work, don't give up. Try something else; modify your short-term plans so that your steps are easier, give yourself more time to accomplish difficult tasks, choose new steps to your goal, or check with your consultants for advice and assistance.

1. The first and most important step is to *identify the problem*. This is usually the most difficult step as well. You may know, for example, that stairs are a problem for you, but it will take a little more effort to determine that the real problem is fear of falling.

2. Once you have identified the problem, the next step is to *list ideas to solve the problem*. You may be able to come up with a good list yourself, but often calling in help from consultants is helpful. Consultants can be friends, family, members of your health care team, or community resources.

3. When you have a list of ideas, *pick one to try*. As you try something new, remember that new activities are usually difficult. Be sure to give your potential solution a fair chance before deciding it won't work.

4. After you've given your idea a fair trial, assess the results. Was the idea helpful? If all has gone well, your problem will be solved.

5. If you still have the problem, choose another idea from your list and try again.

Problem-Solving Steps

1. Identify the problem (this is the most difficult and most important step).

2. List ideas to solve the problem.

3. Select one method to try.

4. Assess the results.

5. Substitute another idea if the first didn't work.

6. Utilize other resources (ask friends, family, professionals for your ideas if your solutions didn't work).

7. Accept that the problem may not be solvable now.

---

6. If a solution still eludes you, *utilize other resources* (your consultants) for more ideas.

7. If all of the above steps do not work, you may have to *accept that your problem may not be solvable right now.* This is sometimes hard to do. However, just because a problem is not solvable right now doesn't mean that it won't be solvable later or that other problems can't be solved in the same way. Even if your path is blocked, there are probably alternate paths. Don't give up. Keep going.

Rewarding Yourself

The best part of being a good self-manager is the rewards you will receive in accomplishing your goals and in living a fuller and more comfortable life. However, don't wait until your goal is reached—reward yourself frequently. For example, decide that you won't read the paper until after you exercise. Reading the paper then becomes your reward. One self-manager rewards himself with ice cream from a café after finishing each of his medical appointments. Another self-manager who stopped smoking used the money he would have spent on cigarettes to have his house professionally cleaned, and there was even enough left over to go to a baseball game with a friend. Rewards don't have to be fancy, expensive, or unhealthy. There are many healthy pleasures that can add enjoyment to your life.

One last note: Not all goals are achievable. Chronic illness may mean having to give up some options. If this is true for you, don't dwell too much on

The Successful Self-Manager
• Sets goals
• Makes a list of alternatives for reaching the goal
• Makes short-term plans or contracts toward that goal
• Carries out the contract
• Checks on progress weekly
• Makes midcourse changes as necessary
• Uses rewards for a job well done

what you can't do. Rather, start working on another goal you would like to accomplish. One self-manager we know who uses a wheelchair talks about the 90 percent of things he *can* do. He spends his life developing this 90 percent to the fullest.

Now that you understand the meaning of self-management, you are ready to begin using the tools that will make you a self-manager. Chapter 13 gives some basic information about HIV and AIDS. Chapters 3 and 4 contain information on some of the common chronic symptoms with HIV. In Chapter 12, we talk about medications and their uses. The rest of the book is devoted to tools of the trade. These include exercise, nutrition, symptom management, communication, making decisions about the future, finding resources, and information about the durable power of attorney for health care.

Contract Form

In writing your contract, be sure it includes:

- *What* you are going to do
- *How much* you are going to do
- *When* you are going to do it
- *How many* days a week you are going to do it

For example: This week, I will walk (*what*) around the block (*how much*) before lunch (*when*) three times (*how many*).

This week I will _____ (*what*)

_____ (*how much*)

_____ (*when*)

_____ (*how many*)

How confident are you that you can complete this contract? _____

(Write a number between 0 and 10, where 0 = not at all confident, 10 = totally confident.)

	Check off	Comments
Monday		
Tuesday		
Wednesday		
Thursday		
Friday		
Saturday		
Sunday		

PART

2

Managing
Symptoms

3

Evaluating Common
Symptoms of HIV/AIDS

▬

Symptoms are the body's signals that something unusual is happening, that something is not right. They cannot always be seen by others, are often difficult to describe, and are usually unpredictable. Having HIV/AIDS means that you are probably going to have symptoms that will need to be managed. Although some symptoms are common, when and how they affect us is very personal. Also, symptoms such as fatigue, stress, shortness of breath, pain, anger, depression, and sleep disturbances can interact with each other, which in turn worsens health and leads to the development of new symptoms.

Although the chronic symptoms of HIV/AIDS are difficult to live with, there are many things you can learn to deal with them better. In this chapter we will look at how to evaluate some of the common symptoms associated with HIV/AIDS to help you decide whether a symptom needs immediate medical attention. If you have not experienced any symptoms yet, this information will help you prepare for what to expect if symptoms do begin. It will also help you determine when symptoms are part of a normal illness, such as a common cold or the flu, or the beginning of the more serious, chronic problems associated with HIV/AIDS. In Chapter 4, we will discuss the more common chronic symptoms of HIV/AIDS and some of their different causes, and in Chapter 5 we will present some specific suggestions for dealing with these symptoms, particularly those techniques that involve the use of the mind.

In addition to helping you deal with your disease symptoms, the various techniques described throughout the book will also help you to maintain health or to slow or prevent the onset of some symptoms.

Keep the following suggestions in mind when trying out a self-management technique and planning your self-management program:

- *Read all three chapters on symptoms and their management* (Chapters 3–5).

- *Evaluate each new symptom.* Symptoms are always distressing, but sometimes they are important clues that something new is happening that needs to be addressed. A new or worsening symptom could be a sign of an opportunistic infection.* To be a good self-manager, you need to know when it's okay to use home self-management techniques and when you should see the doctor.

- *Pick one technique to try first.* Be sure to give this method a fair trial. We recommend that you practice it for at least two weeks, twice a day, before deciding whether the technique is going to be helpful to you. Also, try some of the other techniques, giving each the same trial period. It is important to try more than one technique because some may be more useful for a particular symptom or you may find that you simply prefer some techniques over others.

- *After choosing the techniques you like, think about how and when you will use each one.* This will depend on exactly what you're trying to accomplish. Some techniques are specific for certain symptoms—for example, certain diet changes may be appropriate for managing diarrhea, whereas inhaling moist heat is good for nasal congestion. Some of the exercises can be done anywhere, whereas others require a quiet place. Others may require substantial lifestyle changes. Also, you may find in your practice of the different techniques that some work better to manage specific symptoms and not so well for others. The best symptom-managers learn to use a variety of techniques tailored to their needs and situations on a daily basis.

- *Finally, because practice and consistency are important for the mastery of some of these techniques, place cues in your environment to remind you to practice them.* For example, place a sticker or note where you'll see it, such as on your mirror, in your office, next to your medicines, on the car's dashboard, or near your home phone. You can change the stickers or notes periodically so you will continue to notice them. Also, try linking these new activities to some other established behavior or activity in your daily routine. For example, practice relaxation as part of your cooldown from exercise. You might ask a friend, family member, or partner to remind you to get your practice in each day; they may even wish to participate.

---

* "Opportunistic infection" is a general term for all the serious infections associated with HIV.

Evaluating Your Symptoms

One of the distressing things about living with HIV is that one is always concerned about developing an AIDS-related infection or other condition. New symptoms, especially if they are your first symptoms, are distressing in and of themselves, and also because they could be signals of a new or more serious problem. The truth is that sometimes symptoms *can* be signals that a serious illness is starting and you should see your doctor. Just as often, however, the symptoms are part of the vicious cycle of chronic disease, for which self-management may be the best thing to try.

To feel confident in using self-management, you need to know when it's time to call the doctor. But how can you tell? Some of it is common sense. If it's clear you're having a medical emergency, see a doctor immediately. On the other hand, if you're having symptoms similar to what you've often had in the past, you can probably use self-management techniques confidently.

Another important factor is knowing your T cell count (also called CD4 cell count). T cells are one way of estimating the strength of the immune system; people with a T-cell count lower than 200 are usually at higher risk for getting infections, so they have to be more careful. Your doctor should measure your T cell count at least every six months, and it's a good idea to know the result of your most recent measurement. Of course, T cells aren't the only measure of how healthy you are—or even the most important. But they are useful. There's more information about T cells in Chapter 13.

One quick way to judge whether you should see a doctor for a symptom is to do a FAST check. Ask yourself the four simple questions listed in the chart below. If the answer to any of the questions is *yes*, you should see your doctor promptly. He or she will be able to tell you if the symptom is due to a new AIDS-related infection or cancer.

Do a FAST Check on All New or Worsening Symptoms	
Fever	Is the new symptom associated with a fever (a temperature of 101°F or more)?
Altered Mental Status	Is the new symptom associated with alteration in mental status (confusion, sleepiness, seizures)?
Severe	Is the new symptom much more severe than anything you've had in the past?
Typical	Is the new symptom *not* typical for you?

Fever

Fever can be a chronic symptom in HIV/AIDS, but it also can be an important clue when it appears in association with another symptom. A temperature of 101°F (38.3°C) is more likely to be associated with infection.

Note: *Everyone* with HIV needs to own, and know how to use, a thermometer. It is important to *measure* your temperature when you think you have a fever. *Write down* the temperature, so you will be able to tell the doctor if necessary.

Altered Mental Status

The brain is the body's most important organ, so it is a sensitive indicator of when trouble is present. *Altered mental status* is a term doctors use to describe a person whose brain functioning is not normal. This can mean confusion, excessive sleepiness, or "I can't put my finger on it, but he just isn't himself." It can also be much more dramatic, like a coma (the most extreme decrease in mental function) or a seizure. All of these represent altered mental status. Anyone who develops new altered mental status, particularly in association with other symptoms, should see a doctor promptly.

If you have a serious alteration in mental function, you may not be able to recognize the problem yourself, but you can teach those close to you how to easily diagnose such a change. If they suspect you may be having an altered mental status, they should simply see how you answer questions. If you can't answer questions coherently or can't wake up enough to answer them, urgent action is needed.

Severe

Chronic symptoms will often increase and decrease depending on whether you're having a good day, or a bad day. However, any symptom that is much more severe than it has ever been before should be evaluated by your health care team.

Typical

Any symptom that is completely new for you (that is *not typical*), should be discussed with your medical team. This is a very general guideline that you probably use already when deciding whether to go to the doctor. Depending on what the new symptom is, you may want to consult one of the symptom action charts that follow for more guidance. But remember that when in doubt, it's better to be safe than sorry. If you're experiencing a symptom you've never had before and you're not sure whether self-care is the right thing to do, it's best to consult your doctor to be sure.

Using Symptom Action Charts

Another way to evaluate your symptoms is to use an action chart. These charts will help guide you in evaluating several common HIV/AIDS-related symptoms that sometimes require a doctor's rapid attention. Not every symptom is included, but if you have one of the symptoms listed, the chart will help you decide what to do.

If you have more than one symptom, you may need to look at more than one chart. If the advice doesn't agree between the two charts, follow the most "conservative" (that is, the safest) advice. For example, if one chart says to call the doctor and the other recommends home treatment, you should call your doctor.

If you use the charts properly by following the steps below, they will guide you through the key questions you should consider in deciding whether you need the help of your health care team right away:

1. *Determine your "chief complaint"* or symptom, then find the correct chart. (They are arranged alphabetically.)

2. Before you look at the chart, *read the general information* on the symptom opposite the chart. This information will help you understand the questions in the chart. If you ignore the general information, you may not understand the questions in the chart correctly, and you could do the wrong thing.

3. *Read the action chart.* Start at the top and follow the arrows. Skipping around may result in errors. Each question assumes that you have answered all of the previous questions.

Note: These charts are only intended to help you decide if you need to see your doctor urgently for certain symptoms. Regardless of symptoms, you should always go to the routine check-ups that you and your doctor have scheduled.

Cough

The *cough reflex* is a defense mechanism used by the body to expel abnormal material from the lungs. When the cough is expelling infected material, such as pus, from the lungs, coughing is beneficial and shouldn't be suppressed. However, anything that irritates the lungs will cause a cough, and many of these stimuli do not produce pus, or even anything that's particularly easy to get out. So the cough will continue but not produce anything, and it can be quite aggravating.

People with HIV/AIDS get coughs for all the same reasons other people do. Smoking is probably the most common cause—the toxins in the smoke irritate and kill cells in the linings of the *bronchial tubes* (breathing tubes) and stimulate the cough. This can happen even to those who don't smoke themselves, but who breathe other people's smoke. Viral infections ("colds") are the next most common cause. These coughs usually produce only yellow or whitish mucus, not the green or rusty stuff produced by a more serious bacterial infection. Cold viruses don't respond to antibiotics; the only treatment is to strengthen the body's immune response with rest, good food, and lots of fluids. Bacterial infections can be more serious and require a doctor's attention and antibiotics.

In addition to the usual causes of cough, people with HIV/AIDS are susceptible to lung diseases not usually seen in people with stronger immune systems. The most common and most important of these is *Pneumocystis carinii* pneumonia (PCP). Identifying this disease early is vital because it is very dangerous when advanced. When caught early, however, it responds very well to antibiotics. The signs of PCP are a *dry cough* with *shortness of breath* and *fever*. Other lung infections that are also seen in HIV/AIDS include tuberculosis (TB) and bacterial pneumonia. TB is a very serious lung disease that may cause a chronic cough with fevers but which may not cause much trouble breathing. Unfortunately, TB is very easy to pass on to other people by coughing. Because of the risk of TB, you ought to bring any persistent cough (longer than ten days) to the attention of your doctor.

Infection in the sinuses (*sinusitis*) doesn't affect the lungs directly, but it often causes cough because mucus from the sinuses drips down the throat into the lungs, irritating them. This is particularly a problem at night.

Continued on page 32

COUGH		**Action Chart**

Is the cough associated with *shortness of breath at rest*, or with *minimal exertion?* → Yes → See doctor now

↓ No

Is the cough *dry*, and associated with *fever?* → Yes → See doctor today

↓ No

Is the cough associated with *fever* and *pain in the chest?* → Yes → See doctor today

↓ No

Is the cough producing thick, foul-smelling *rusty or greenish mucus?* → Yes → See doctor today

↓ No

Has *fever* lasted for more than 4 days or has cough persisted for more than 10 days? → Yes → Make appointment with doctor

↓ No

Home treatment (see page 32)

Cough, continued

Home Treatment of Cough

The mucus in the bronchial tubes may be made thinner and less sticky by several means. Increasing the humidity in the air will help; a vaporizer and a steamy shower are two ways to add humidity. Drinking large quantities of fluid is helpful for cough, particularly if a fever has dehydrated the body. Glyceryl guaiacolate (Robitussin) may help liquify the secretions so they can be coughed out of the lungs more easily; it won't suppress the cough, however. Decongestants (Sudafed) and/or antihistamines (Benadryl) may help if the cough is caused by nasal or sinus material dripping down into the lungs. (**Note:** These medicines should otherwise be avoided because they dry the secretions and make them thicker.*)

Dry, tickling coughs are often relieved by cough lozenges or sucking on hard candy. Dextromethorphan (Robitussin-DM) is an effective cough suppressant available without a prescription, but neither this nor codeine (available only with a prescription) will completely eliminate cough, even at high dosage.

Diarrhea

Many of the concerns with diarrhea are the same as those with nausea and vomiting. *Dehydration* is the greatest risk and can require intravenous medicines when it gets severe. Diarrhea that is *jet black* or *bloody* may indicate significant bleeding from the intestines. Most people with diarrhea will have cramping, intermittent gas-like pains, but *severe, steady abdominal pain* could be more serious. In people with HIV/AIDS, diarrhea can be caused by viral, bacterial, or parasitic infections and is often caused by the effect of HIV itself on the intestines. Medications may also be the culprit; people with HIV/AIDS often use antibiotics, ddI, or anticancer drugs, all of which may cause diarrhea. If medications may be responsible, call the prescribing doctor.

---

*Over-the-counter cold medicines almost always contain antihistamine—and/or decongestant and/or expectorant—in some bewildering combination or another.

DIARRHEA		*Action Chart*

Are *either* of the following present?   Yes   See doctor
- *black or bloody stools*   ➡   now
- *severe, steady abdominal pain*

⬇ No

Do you have any signs of dehydration?   Yes   See doctor
- *extreme thirst*   • *very dry mouth*   ➡   today
- *dark urine*   • *lightheadedness*

⬇ No

Are you taking *antibiotics?*   Yes   Call doctor
                                        ➡

⬇ No

Had *diarrhea* been severe for longer   Yes   Call
than 5 days without improvement?   ➡   doctor

⬇ No

Home treatment (see below)

Home Treatment of Diarrhea

Home treatment of diarrhea is directed at getting adequate fluid into the body to prevent dehydration. Sip clear fluids, such as water or ginger ale. If you are vomiting and nothing else will stay down, suck on ice chips—this is usually tolerated and provides some fluids. Gatorade, bouillon, and Jell-O are also good sources of liquid. The next step is to move on to constipating foods: the "BRAT" diet of bananas, rice, applesauce, and toast. Milk and fats will not absorb well and should be avoided for a few days. Nonprescription preparations such as Kaopectate will change the stool to a semisolid state, but they won't change the amount or frequency of the stools. Many cases of diarrhea will resolve on their own within 5 days, but if this doesn't happen, you may need evaluation and should call your doctor. You may eventually need stronger medication to slow down the intestinal tract.

Fever

The most common cause of fevers in HIV/AIDS is infection. Probably the single most common cause of fever is HIV itself. Fever can be due to viral, bacterial, and parasitic infections and sometimes is due to cancers or medications. Fever is a distressing symptom, but it's rarely dangerous in itself. However, the infection that might be causing the fever could be very serious. Everyone needs to know how to measure a fever and how to decide when the fever needs to be evaluated right away.

Everyone with HIV must have a thermometer and know how to use it properly. Both Fahrenheit and Centigrade thermometers are okay. If the temperature is greater than or equal to 101°F, it's important to consider whether one of the serious, emergency AIDS-associated infections could be present. These include meningitis, an infection of the lining of the brain that causes *neck stiffness* and *confusion*, and *Pneumocystis* pneumonia, an infection of the lungs that causes *dry cough* and *shortness of breath*, particularly on exertion. People with a permanent central intravenous (IV) line (usually inserted into the upper arm or the chest) are at risk for bacterial sepsis (blood poisoning) and should be evaluated promptly for *new fevers*.

If none of these problems is present, the fever still could be serious but probably doesn't require immediate attention by a doctor. The important consideration is what symptoms are associated with the fever, and how they should be managed.

Home Treatment of Fever

There are two ways to reduce a fever: sponging and medication. Sponging the skin with tepid water will bring the body temperature down as the water evaporates. Medications to lower fever include aspirin, acetaminophen (Tylenol, Datril), and ibuprofen (Motrin, Advil). Adults can take two aspirin every 3 to 4 hours as required. Acetaminophen is taken similarly and is often confused with aspirin, but it is a completely different medicine. It has the same effect as aspirin on lowering the temperature but causes less stomach upset. On the other hand, overdoses of acetaminophen can be fatal, and it can cause liver damage in high doses. Since aspirin and acetaminophen are different drugs, they can be given together to control temperature when one or the other alone is not effective. To do this, stagger the doses every 3 hours, alternating doses of aspirin and acetaminophen.

FEVER   *Action Chart*

Is your temperature greater than or equal to 101°F (38.3°C) and associated with
- *neck stiffness?*
- *lethargy or confusion?*
- *seizure?*
- *severe irritability?*

Yes → See doctor now

↓ No

Is your temperature greater than or equal to 101°F (38.3°C) and associated with *dry cough and severe shortness of breath?*

Yes → See doctor now

↓ No

Is this a *new fever* in a person with a central IV (intravenous) line for medications?

Yes → Call or see doctor today

↓ No

Is the *fever* associated with a new *skin rash* or *skin sores?*

Yes → Call or see doctor today

↓ No

Is the *fever* associated with
- *headache?*   • *sore throat?*
- *cough* (not short   • *diarrhea?*
  of breath)?   • *urinary problems?*

Yes → See section on the associated problem

↓ No

Home treatment (see opposite)

Headache

Headache is the single most frequent complaint of modern times. The most common causes of headache are tension (something that people with HIV/AIDS often have) and muscle spasms. Medications can also lead to headaches; Zidovudine (AZT) is a frequent cause for some people.

However, there are several important opportunistic diseases that can start out as headaches in people with HIV/AIDS. Headache associated with *fever* and a *neck so stiff that the chin cannot be touched to the chest* suggests the possibility of meningitis, a serious infection of the lining of the brain. Headaches could be caused by infection or tumor in the brain itself if they are associated with neurological problems such as *slurred speech, weakness or paralysis in the arms or the legs,* or new *visual problems.* And any headache that comes after a *severe head injury* could be serious.

Home Treatment of Headache

The usual over-the-counter drugs (aspirin, acetaminophen, ibuprofen) are quite effective in relieving headache. Headache also responds very well to techniques directed at reducing stress and tension. It is frequently relieved by massage or heat applied to the back of the upper neck or by simply resting with the eyes closed and the head supported. Meditation is often effective. Headaches that don't respond to these measures should be brought to the attention of a doctor.

HEADACHE — *Action Chart*

Is the headache associated with *fever* greater than or equal to 101°F (38.3°C) and *neck stiffness?*   Yes ⟶ See doctor now

↓ No

Is the headache associated with
- *problems moving arms or legs?*
- *vision problems?*
- *slurred speech?*
- *recent head injury?*

Yes ⟶ See doctor today

↓ No

Has the headache lasted less than 3 days?   Yes ⟶ Home treatment (see opposite)

↓ No

Home treatment (see opposite) and make appointment with doctor

Impaired/Decreased Vision

Your vision is important, so any vision change should lead you to see the doctor if it doesn't improve on its own. The most common causes of vision problems in people with HIV/AIDS are not different than in other people: nearsightedness and farsightedness. Also, sometimes vision will be affected by medications, headaches, eye strain, or fatigue. When one of these things is causing vision problems, the change is usually gradual and about equal in both eyes. Your condition should certainly be evaluated, but it isn't an emergency. But HIV/AIDS also can lead to CMV (cytomegalovirus) retinitis, an infection of the back of the eye (retina) that can damage the visual field severely. In its worst forms, CMV retinitis can lead to blindness, but it can be arrested with medications. This is why you should see the doctor for any visual change, and you should see him or her promptly about a rapid or asymmetric visual change.

Home Treatment of Impaired/Decreased Vision

If you experience temporary changes in your vision caused by medications or fatigue, try resting with your eyes closed in a darkened room for a few minutes. On bright days, be sure to protect your eyes with sunglasses; this will decrease strain and allow your eyes to accommodate more easily. Permanent changes in your vision should be discussed with your doctor.

IMPAIRED/DECREASED VISION   *Action Chart*

Did *blindness* (partial or complete) occur *suddenly* in one or both eyes or is the *visual loss severe?*   → Yes → See doctor now

↓ No

Is your *T cell count* (CD4 cell count) *over 200?*   Yes → Make appointment with doctor

↓ No

Have you had *gradual vision loss about equal* in both eyes?   Yes → Make appointment with doctor

↓ No

See doctor today

Nausea and Vomiting

Many of the concerns with nausea and vomiting are the same as those with diarrhea. Medications are the most common cause of nausea in people with HIV/AIDS, although viral infections can also cause problems. *Dehydration* is the greatest risk; as with diarrhea, intravenous medicines may be needed when it gets severe. People with severe dehydration often have dizziness, severe thirst, dry mouth and tongue, decreased amounts of urine, dark urine, and wrinkled dry skin. *Vomit that is bloody or black* may indicate that severe intestinal bleeding is present. This problem is particularly bad in people with liver disease. Sometimes an infection of the brain can lead to nausea and vomiting, so if you have a *headache* and a *stiff neck*, you should see your doctor right away. Women who are sexually active should always consider the possibility that their nausea is due to pregnancy. The best way to know for sure is to get a pregnancy test, either over the counter at your local drugstore or in your doctor's office.

Many medications used in HIV/AIDS care can cause nausea. Antibiotics and anticancer drugs are two examples, but there are many, many others. If nausea begins soon after you start a *new medicine*, call the doctor.

Home Treatment of Nausea and Vomiting

The objective of home treatment of nausea is to get as much fluid as possible into your body without upsetting your stomach any further. Sip clear fluids, such as water or ginger ale. Suck on ice chips if nothing else will stay down. Don't drink too much at any one time as this will aggravate the stomach. Add Gatorade, bouillon, soups, and Jell-O as your condition improves. If the vomiting does not resolve within 3 days, call the doctor.

| **NAUSEA AND VOMITING** | | **Action Chart** |

Are *any* of the following present?   Yes   ⟶   See doctor now
- *black or bloody vomit*
- *severe, steady abdominal pain*
- *headache and stiff neck*

↓ No

Do you have any signs of dehydration?   Yes   ⟶   See doctor today
- *extreme thirst*   • *very dry mouth*
- *dark urine*   • *lightheadedness*

↓ No

Did this begin after starting a *new medication?*   Yes   ⟶   Call doctor

↓ No

Are you *pregnant,* or do you think you might be pregnant?   Yes   ⟶   Call doctor

↓ No

Have you been *vomiting* longer than 3 days without improvement?   Yes   ⟶   Call doctor

↓ No

Home treatment (see opposite)

Shortness of Breath

Shortness of breath is normal under circumstances of strenuous activity. But if you get "winded" at rest or with only minimal exertion, or if you wake up at night short of breath, you have a serious symptom that should be evaluated promptly by a doctor. In people with HIV/AIDS, the major concern is pneumonia, most often caused by *Pneumocystis carinii*. *Pneumocystis* almost always causes a dry cough and a fever, so these symptoms are very important. Everyone must have a working thermometer and know how to use it!

There are several other causes of chronic shortness of breath, including lung damage caused by previous lung infections, anemia, and smoking-induced lung disease. These are described in Chapter 4, along with some self-management techniques that may be helpful.

Home Treatment of Shortness of Breath

Several suggestions about things that are often helpful for people with shortness of breath are given in Chapter 4 of this book.

SHORTNESS OF BREATH   *Action Chart*

Do you have *shortness of breath at rest*, or with *minimal exertion?*   Yes   ⟶   See doctor now

↓ No

Is the shortness of breath associated with *dry cough* and *fever?*   Yes   ⟶   See doctor now

↓ No

Home treatment (see Chapter 4) and make appointment with doctor

Sore Throat

Sore throat is almost never a life-threatening problem, but it can be painful. Sore throats can be caused by several infections. "Cold" viruses are the most common cause and cannot be treated successfully with antibiotics; they must run their course. Mononucleosis ("mono") is a viral infection that causes a more severe, prolonged illness with painful swelling and soreness in the throat. Even though it sounds formidable, "mono" rarely causes complications and usually gets better with rest. Again, antibiotics don't treat mononucleosis.

Streptococcal bacteria ("strep throat") are another common cause of sore throat. These should be treated with antibiotics in order to prevent the small chance of an abscess forming and to prevent the secondary damage to the kidneys that can sometimes occur. It's hard to tell when a sore throat might be "strep throat," but it's unlikely if the sore throat is a minor part of a typical cold (runny nose, stuffy ears, etc.). A high temperature, pus in the back of the throat, or swollen tonsils can be clues indicating strep throat might be present. Sore throat in people with HIV/AIDS can also be caused by infection with candida (thrush) or by ulcers in the throat from herpes or CMV (cytomegalovirus) infections.

None of these conditions are emergencies (unless, of course, *you are unable to eat or breathe*), but they should be looked at by a doctor. Therefore, if your sore throat doesn't seem to be associated with usual "cold" symptoms, or if it lasts for longer than 10 days, you should contact your doctor.

Home Treatment of Sore Throat

Cold liquids, aspirin, ibuprofen, and acetaminophen are effective for the pain and fever. If you have had oral thrush in the past and think you might have it now (white, cottage cheese-like material in your mouth), you should start the thrush medicine your doctor gave you (usually clotrimazole [Mycelex] "troches"). Home remedies that may help include salt water gargles and honey or lemon in tea.

SORE THROAT   *Action Chart*

Do you have *severe difficulty swallow-*
ing or *difficulty breathing?*   Yes ⟶   See doctor
                                                    now

↓ No

Are *either* of the following condi-
tions present?   Yes ⟶   Call the doctor
• *temperature of 101°F or more*   today
• *pus in the back of the throat*

↓ No

Are your *tonsils swollen?*   Yes ⟶   Obtain a
                                                    throat culture

↓ No

Has your sore throat *lasted longer*
than 10 days?   Yes ⟶   Call the doctor
                                                    today

↓ No

Home treatment (see opposite)

Urination Problems—Painful, Frequent, or Bloody Urination

Urinary infections are much more common in women than in men, but men can sometimes get them, especially in the setting of HIV/AIDS. The most common symptoms of urinary infection are *pain or burning on urination, frequent urgent urination, and blood in the urine.* But sometimes these symptoms are not caused by infection. They can also be due to excessive use of caffeine-containing beverages (coffee, tea, or cola), bladder spasms, or even anxiety. Bladder infection in women is often caused by sexual activity.

If *fever, vomiting, back pain,* or *teeth-chattering or body-shaking chills* are present, this suggests that the infection may have spread from the bladder to the kidneys and is much more serious. Bladder infections are common during *pregnancy,* and the treatment is more difficult. For women that get repeated bladder infections, it is important to remember to wipe the toilet tissue from front to back after urinating. Most bacteria that cause bladder infections come from the rectum.

Home Treatment of Urination Problems

Home treatment depends on drinking a lot of fluids. Increase fluid intake to as much as several gallons of fluid in the first 24 hours after symptoms start. Bacteria are literally washed out of the body with the resulting urination. Drink fruit juices to put more acid into the urine; cranberry juice is the most effective, since it contains a natural antibiotic. Begin home treatment as soon as you notice the symptoms. Relief may well begin before you see the doctor.

Sometimes irritation from the vagina can cause frequent urination or blood in the urine. When this happens, the infection may not be in the urinary system, but in the vagina or cervix. If there is *pain in the abdomen* along with *vaginal discharge,* this suggests a serious disease, ranging from gonorrhea to an ectopic pregnancy in the fallopian tube. These things are also suggested by *bloody discharge* that comes between periods and is frequent or in large amounts. All these conditions should be evaluated by the doctor. Candida yeast (the same thing that causes thrush) often causes discharge from the vagina—it looks like white, cheesy material. It may respond to over-the-counter antiyeast medications (Monistat, Mycolog), but some women with HIV/AIDS need stronger medicines available only by prescription.

The major concern in women with discharge from the vagina is the possibility of sexually transmitted disease (STD). All the organisms that cause STDs can cause severe infections in women with HIV/AIDS. If sexual contact

| URINATION PROBLEMS | | Action Chart |

Are the symptoms (painful, frequent, or bloody urination) associated with *fever, vomiting, back pain,* or *shaking chills* or is there a chance you could be *pregnant?* → **Yes** → See doctor today

↓ **No**

Is the problem associated with a new, irritating *vaginal discharge?* → **Yes** → Is the *vaginal discharge* associated with *pain in the abdomen?*

↓ **No**

Home treatment (see opposite) and call the doctor today

↓ **No**

Home treatment (see opposite)

↓ **Yes**

See doctor today

in the past few weeks might possibly have led to an STD, the doctor *must* be seen. It's okay to start home self-management, but make an appointment with the doctor, too.

Women who are taking antibiotics often get worse yeast infections in the vagina. To prevent these infections, it's helpful to eat yogurt, buttermilk, or sour cream and to use less sugar and alcohol. It may be helpful to call the doctor for advice on changing the medication.

Suggested Reading

Vickery, Donald M., and James F. Fries. *Take Care of Yourself.* Reading, Mass.: Addison-Wesley, 1989.

4

Understanding Common Symptoms of HIV/AIDS

Knowing how to evaluate symptoms is only part of what's necessary to become a good self-manager. By better understanding the *causes* of your symptoms, you can better identify ways to deal with the causes, and you can help prevent the symptoms from recurring. Understanding symptoms and their causes better is what this chapter is all about. We won't cover every single symptom a person with HIV/AIDS might get—there are too many of them—but we will cover some of the major symptoms that appear chronically in many people. Many of these symptoms (like fatigue, stress, anger, and sleeping problems) are not things that are easily treatable with medications, so doctors often don't deal with them very well.

It may seem as though it should be easy to identify what symptoms are bothering you and what the cause of each symptom is, but remember that the symptoms and problems associated with HIV/AIDS can be numerous, complex, and interrelated. Imagine that each cause and each symptom have their own threads; for every symptom, then, you may have two or more threads. Then you add more threads for each way in which the symptom affects your life. When you have more than one symptom with two or more causes interacting in your daily life, these threads can become very tangled. To successfully manage your symptoms, you must figure out how to untangle these threads. You may overhear someone saying, "Oh, I know *exactly* what you mean. I had that same problem. All I had to do was . . . and I was as good as new!" Although you may be tempted to believe this person, in fact he or she may not understand *exactly* what you mean and how this symptom is affecting *your* life. We are all unique, and how HIV/AIDS affects each person is also unique.

As you read this chapter you will notice that some symptoms have the same causes. Sometimes a symptom may cause another symptom. The idea is to gain an understanding about the causes of *your* symptoms and to learn to deal with them better.

Anger—Why Me?

Anger is one of the most common responses to having HIV/AIDS. The uncertainty and unpredictability of living with HIV/AIDS threatens what you have fought all your life to achieve—independence and control. The loss of control over your body and loss of independence in life create feelings of frustration, helplessness, and hopelessness, all of which fuel the anger. In fact, at various times during the course of your illness, you may find yourself asking, "Why me?" You may wonder what you did to deserve this, or why you are being punished. All of these are normal anger responses to HIV/AIDS.

You may be angry with yourself, your partner, family, friends, health care providers, God, or the world in general—all for a variety of reasons. You may be angry at yourself for becoming HIV-infected in the first place. You may be angry at your partner, family, and friends because they don't do things the way you would like them done. You may be angry at your doctor because he or she cannot "fix" you. Other people's attitudes about you and this disease may also anger you. Sometimes your anger may be misplaced, as when you find yourself yelling at the cat or dog. Misplaced anger is quite common, especially if you are not even aware that you are angry or why.

Sometimes the anger is not just a response to having a chronic illness but is actually the result of the disease process itself. For example, if you have suffered a brain infection that has affected a certain part of the brain, your ability to express or suppress emotions may be affected. Some people who have had brain infections may thus appear to cry inappropriately or have flares in temper.

Recognizing (or admitting) that you are angry and identifying why, or with whom, are important in learning how to manage your anger effectively. This task also involves finding constructive ways to express your anger. If not expressed, the anger becomes unhealthy. It can build up until it becomes explosive and offends others or is turned inward, thereby intensifying the experience of other disease symptoms, such as depression.

Dealing with Anger

There are several things that you can do to help manage your anger:

- *Learn how to communicate your anger verbally,* preferably without blaming or offending others. (Using "I" messages rather than "you" messages to express your feelings will help you avoid blaming—these are discussed more fully in Chapter 10.) However, if you choose to express your anger verbally, know that many people will not be able to help you. Most of us are not very good at, or comfortable with, dealing with angry people, even if the anger is justified. Therefore, you may also find it useful to seek counseling or join a support group. Voluntary organizations, such as your local AIDS foundation, may be useful resources in this area.

- *Modify your expectations.* You have done this throughout your life. For example, as a child you thought you could become anything—a fire-fighter, a ballet dancer, a doctor. As you grew older, however, you reevaluated these expectations, along with your capabilities, talents, and interests. From this reevaluation, you modified your plans. You can use this same process to deal with the effects of HIV/AIDS on your life. For example, it may be unrealistic to expect that you will get "all better." However, it is realistic to expect that you can still do many pleasurable things. You have the ability to affect the progress of your illness by slowing its decline or preventing it from becoming worse. Changing your expectations can help you to change your perspective. Instead of dwelling on the 10 percent of things you can no longer do, think about the 90 percent of things you still can do. You may even be able to find new activities or hobbies to replace old ones. Learning to think positively or to talk to yourself positively can also help to change your perspective. We discuss this more in Chapter 5.

- *Channel your anger through new activities,* such as exercise, writing, listening to music, or painting. Some people find these extremely therapeutic outlets for angry feelings.

In short, anger is a normal response to having a chronic disease. Part of learning to manage the disease involves acknowledging this anger and finding constructive ways to deal with it.

Depression

Depression can be a frightening word. Some people prefer saying that they are "blue" or "feeling down." Whatever you call it, depression is a normal reaction to chronic illness. Sometimes it is not easy to recognize when you are depressed. Even more difficult is recognizing when you may be becoming depressed and then catching yourself before you fall into a deep depression. Just as there are many degrees of pain, there are many different degrees of depression. If your disease is a significant problem in your life, you almost certainly have, or have had, some problems with depression. Although depression is felt by everyone at some time, it is how you handle it that makes the difference. There are many different signs of depression, which will be discussed later in this section.

Emotions Leading to Depression

Several emotions can lead to depression:

- *Fear, anxiety, and/or uncertainty about the future.* Whether these feelings result from worries about finances, the disease process, your partner, or your family, constant worry about these issues can lead to depression if they are not addressed by you and those involved. In Chapter 15 we discuss some decisions all of us will have to make at some time in our lives. By confronting these issues early on, you will put your mind at rest and have more time to enjoy life.

- *Frustration.* Any number of things can call up feelings of frustration. You may find yourself thinking, "I just can't do what I want," "I feel so helpless," "I used to be able to do this myself," or "Why doesn't anyone understand me?" Feelings like these can leave you feeling more alone and isolated the longer you hold on to them.

- *Loss of control over your life.* Whether it comes from having to rely on medications to ease symptoms; having to see a doctor on a regular basis; or having to count on others to help you perform your daily activities, such as bathing, dressing, and preparing meals, the feeling of losing control can make you lose faith in yourself and your abilities. Your life has suddenly become a team sport in which you are no longer the coach. Instead, you are now a player with someone else calling the plays.

Signs of Depression

- *Loss of interest in friends or activities.* Not wanting to talk to anyone or to answer the phone or doorbell. In short, isolation is an important symptom of depression.
- *Difficulty sleeping*, changed sleeping patterns, interrupted sleep, or sleeping more than usual. You may go to sleep easily but awaken often and be unable to go back to sleep.
- *Changes in eating habits.* This change may range from a loss of interest in food to unusually erratic or excessive eating.
- *Unintentional weight change*, either gain or loss, of more than 10 pounds in a short period of time.
- *Loss of interest in personal care and grooming.*
- *A general feeling of unhappiness* lasting longer than 6 weeks.
- *Loss of interest in being held or in sex.* These problems can sometimes also be due to medication side effects, so it is important that you talk them over with your doctor.
- *Suicidal thoughts.* If your unhappiness has caused you to think about killing yourself, get some help from your doctor, good friends, a member of the clergy, a psychologist, or a social worker. These feelings will pass and you will feel better, so get help and don't let a tragedy happen to you and your loved ones.
- *Frequent accidents.* Watch for a pattern of increased carelessness, accidents while walking or driving, dropping things, and so forth. Of course you must take into account how much the physical problems caused by your disease, such as unsteady balance or slowed reaction times, may be contributing to these incidents.
- *Low self-image.* A feeling of worthlessness, a negative image of your body, wondering if it is all worth it.
- *Frequent arguments.* A tendency to blow up easily over minor matters, over things that never bothered you before.
- *Loss of energy.* Fatigue, feeling tired all the time.
- *Inability to make decisions.* Feeling confused and unable to concentrate.

Although these feelings have been listed separately, they are often experienced in combination, making it more difficult to determine what is really at the root of the depression. Also, we often do not recognize when we are depressed, or do not wish to admit to ourselves that we are actually depressed. Learning to recognize the signs of depression is the first step in learning how to manage it.

Dealing with Depression

It is undeniable that having HIV/AIDS can be very depressing. We would not try to tell you that you should not have feelings of depression about your illness. However, just as the physical deconditioning that happens as a result of HIV/AIDS can make you feel weak and helpless, leading to less physical activity and even more deconditioning, depression can be a vicious cycle of emotional "deconditioning." Depression can cause you to feel helpless and hopeless and to let go of many of your normally pleasurable activities, which in turn makes life seem even more bleak.

Depression makes us see things darkly, and from the standpoint of being depressed, we tend to believe that nothing can be different. Not so! Depression is something that you can manage, just like any other symptom of HIV/AIDS. Part of being very depressed, however, is that you may not be able to dredge up the motivation to get started. You may need to force yourself into action, or to get someone to help you do the things that will help.

Here are some active steps you can take to manage depression:

- *Seek help immediately if you feel like hurting yourself or someone else.* Call your mental health center, doctor, suicide prevention center, a friend, spiritual counselor, or community center. Do not delay. Do it now. Often, just talking with an understanding person or health professional will be enough to help you through this mood.

- *Discontinue tranquilizers or narcotic pain-killers,* such as Valium, Librium, codeine, vicodin, sleeping medications, or other downers. These drugs intensify depression, and the sooner you can stop taking them, the better off you will be. Your depression may be a drug side effect. If you are not sure what you are taking or are uncertain if what you're experiencing could be a side effect, check with a doctor or pharmacist. However, before discontinuing a prescription medication, *always* check, at least by phone, with the prescribing physician, as there may be important reasons for continuing its use or there may be withdrawal reactions.

- *Cut back on drinking alcohol.* Although you may be drinking to feel better, alcohol is also a downer. There is virtually no way to escape depression unless you unload your brain from chemical downers like alcohol. For most people, one or two drinks in the evening is not a problem, but if your mind is not free of alcohol during most of the day, you are having trouble with this drug.

- *Continue your daily activities.* Get dressed every day, make your bed, get out of the house, go shopping, walk your dog. Plan and cook meals. Force yourself to do these things even if you don't feel like it.
- *Visit with friends.* Call them on the phone. Plan to go to the movies or on other outings. Do it!
- *Join a group.* Get involved in a church group, a discussion group at an activity center, a community college class, a self-help class, or a nutrition program.
- *Volunteer.* People who help other people are seldom depressed.
- *Make plans and carry them out.* Look to the future. Plant some young trees. Look forward to some special occasion. If you know that one time of the year is especially difficult, such as Christmas or a birthday, make specific plans for that period. Don't wait to see what happens. Be prepared.
- *Don't move to a new setting* without first visiting for a few weeks. Moving can be a sign of withdrawal, and depression often intensifies when you are in a location away from friends and acquaintances. Troubles usually move with you.
- *Take a vacation* with relatives or friends. Vacations can be as simple as a few days in a nearby city or a resort just a few miles down the road. Rather than go alone, look into trips sponsored by colleges, city recreation departments, the "Y," clubs, support groups, or church groups.
- *Do 20 to 30 minutes of physical exercise every day.*
- *Make a list of self-rewards.* Take care of yourself. You can reward yourself by doing something special for yourself, such as reading at a set time or seeing a special play. Anything, big or small, that you can look forward to during the day, can help combat feelings of depression.
- *If you are very depressed, talk to your doctor or nurse about taking an antidepressant medication.* Such drugs can be very helpful for depression, and one of them may be appropriate for you.

Depression feeds on depression, so *break the cycle.* The success of your self-management program depends on it. Depression is not permanent, and you can hasten its disappearance. Focus on your pride, your friends, your future goals, and your positive surroundings. How you respond to depression is a self-fulfilling prophecy. When you believe that things will get better, they will.

Fatigue

HIV/AIDS can drain your energy. For many people, fatigue is a very real problem and not "all in the mind." It can keep you from doing the things you'd like to do. Furthermore, the effects of fatigue may be misunderstood or underestimated by others. Sometimes family, friends, and partners do not understand the unpredictability of the fatigue associated with HIV/AIDS and may misinterpret it as being a lack of interest in certain activities or as a desire to be alone.

Fatigue can have many causes, including:

- *The disease itself.* When you have HIV/AIDS, activities require more energy. The body is less efficient because some of the energy usually reserved for daily activities is now needed to help the body heal itself.
- *Inactivity.* Muscles not used become deconditioned—that is, they become less efficient at doing what they are supposed to do. The heart, which is made of muscular tissue, can also become deconditioned. When this happens, the heart's ability to pump blood, necessary nutrients, and oxygen to other parts of the body is decreased. When muscles do not receive the nutrients and oxygen necessary to function properly, they tire more easily than do muscles in good condition—the ones that receive an adequate supply of blood, oxygen, and nutrients through physical activity.
- *Poor nutrition.* Food is your basic source of energy. If the fuel you take in is not of top quality and/or in proper quantities, fatigue can result. Malnutrition often results in fatigue, especially for people with HIV/AIDS. Many people with HIV/AIDS experience sudden weight loss because of a change in their eating habits or in their body's use of nutrients.
- *Insufficient rest.* For a variety of reasons, there will be times when you do not get enough sleep or have poor-quality sleep. This can also result in fatigue. The final section of this chapter deals with sleep problems.
- *Emotions.* Stress and depression can also cause significant fatigue. Most people are aware of the connection between stress and feeling tired, but fatigue is also an important symptom of depression.

If fatigue is a problem for you, your first job is to *determine the cause.*

- Are you eating a *proper diet?*
- Are you *exercising?*
- Are you getting enough good-quality *sleep?*

If you answer no to any of these questions, you may be well on your way to determining one or more of the reasons for your fatigue. The important thing to remember about your fatigue is that it may be caused by many things other than your illness. Therefore, in order to fight and prevent fatigue, you must address the cause(s) of your fatigue.

People often say they can't exercise because they feel fatigued. This creates a vicious cycle: you are fatigued because of a lack of exercise, and then you don't exercise because of the fatigue. Believe it or not, if this is your problem, then motivating yourself to do a little *exercise* next time you are fatigued may be the answer. You don't have to run a marathon. Just go outdoors and take a short walk. If this is not possible, then walk around your house. See Chapter 6 for more information on getting started on an exercise program.

If your fatigue is caused by a *poor diet*, such as eating too many empty calories in the form of junk food or alcohol, then the solution is to eat better-quality food as well as proper quantities of food. For some people, the problem may be a decreased interest in food leading to not eating enough and subsequent weight loss. Also, some may not absorb food well due to GI tract problems. Chapters 7, 8, and 9 discuss in greater detail some of the problems associated with eating poorly, as well as tips for improving your eating habits.

If *emotions* are causing your fatigue, rest will not help. In fact, it may make you feel worse. We know that *fatigue is often a sign of depression*, and we discussed ways to deal with depression earlier in this chapter. *Stress* can also cause fatigue; beginning on page 65, we suggest ways to manage it.

Pain

Pain is a problem shared by many people with HIV/AIDS. In fact, it may be their number one concern. As with most symptoms, pain can have many causes.

Common Causes

The four most common causes of pain are:

- *The disease itself.* Pain can come from damaged nerves, swollen internal organs, or irritated skin, just to name a few.
- *Tense muscles.* When something hurts, the muscles in that area become tense. This is your body's natural reaction to pain—to try to protect the damaged area.

- *Muscle deconditioning.* In HIV/AIDS, it is common to become less active, leading to a weakening of the muscles, or muscle deconditioning. When a muscle is weak, it tends to complain anytime it is used. Thus even the slightest activity can sometimes lead to pain and stiffness.
- *Fear and depression.* When you are afraid, frustrated, or depressed, everything, including pain, seems worse. This is not to imply that the pain is not real. Rather, fear and depression tend to make an already bad experience worse.

Because pain comes from many sources, pain management must be aimed at all of these that apply. Medications can help with some disease-caused pain—for example, they can help open blood vessels and bronchial tubes or reduce pain caused by inflammation.

Dealing with Pain

Two of the best ways of dealing with pain are exercise and cognitive pain management techniques, such as relaxation and visualization, in which you actively use your mind to help manage your symptoms. The benefits of exercise, as well as tips for starting an exercise program, are discussed in Chapter 6; using your mind to manage symptoms is discussed in the Chapter 5.

In addition to exercise and cognitive pain management, several other techniques, such as *heat, cold, and massage,* are sometimes useful for localized pain. These three methods work by stimulating the skin and other tissues surrounding the painful area, which increases the blood flow to these areas.

- *Heat.* You can stimulate the blood flow by applying a heating pad or by taking a warm bath or shower (with the water flow directed at the painful area). Limit the application to 15 or 20 minutes at a time.
- *Cold.* Some people prefer cold for soothing the pain. A bag of frozen peas or corn makes an inexpensive, reusable cold pack. Limit the application to 15 or 20 minutes at a time.
- *Massage* is actually one of the oldest forms of pain management. Hippocrates (c. 460–380 B.C.) said that "physicians must be experienced in many things, but assuredly also in the rubbing that can bind a joint that is loose and loosen a joint that is too hard." Self-massage is a simple procedure that can be performed with little practice or preparation. It stimulates the skin, underlying tissues, and muscles by means of applying pressure. Some people like to use a mentholated cream with

self-massage because these creams give a cooling effect. Massage, although relatively simple, is not appropriate for all cases of pain. Do *not* use self-massage for a "hot joint" (one that is red, swollen, and hot to the touch), an infected area, or if you are suffering from phlebitis, thrombophlebitis, or skin eruptions. For more details on specific types of massage, see Suggested Reading at the end of this chapter.

Shortness of Breath

Shortness of breath can be a chronic symptom, or it can be caused by an acute infection that could be dangerous, yet cleared up quite well with proper treatment. To rule out the possibility of an acute infection, be sure to check your symptoms against the Shortness of Breath action chart in Chapter 3 before going on to the things discussed in this section. Shortness of breath, like fatigue and stress, can have many causes. In all cases, your body is not getting the oxygen that it needs. The difference comes in the physiological changes that take place as the result of HIV/AIDS that may lead to an increased sensitivity to different stimuli.

Common Causes

Some of the most common physiological changes taking place as a result of HIV/AIDS and leading to shortness of breath include:

- *Damage to the air sacs* in the lungs, as is the case after some lung infections. Such damage causes the lungs to be less efficient at getting oxygen into the blood and carbon dioxide out. Although the body can adjust to this change to some extent, when there is a sudden change in your "normal" breathing pattern, the lungs cannot always keep up.

- *Narrowing of the airways to the air sacs* and *excess mucus production.* Because the airways become narrowed, there is less room for air to flow through to get to the lungs and thus less oxygen. These changes occur with both asthma and chronic bronchitis. One difference between these two diseases is that with asthma, the narrowing of the airways, along with an increase in mucus production, is in response to some sort of stimulus. The excess mucus production also decreases the amount of space available for the oxygen to get to the lungs.

- *Anemia.* Oxygen is carried in the red blood cells, so people who are anemic (have too few red blood cells) may develop shortness of breath.

- *Deconditioning of muscles.* The deconditioning process can affect the breathing muscles or any of the other muscles in your body. When muscles become deconditioned, they are less efficient in doing what they are supposed to do, so they require more energy (and oxygen) to perform activities than do well-conditioned muscles. In the case of the breathing muscles, clearing the lungs becomes less efficient and less space is left for fresh air to be inhaled.

- *Anxiety and stress.* Anxiety can increase breathing and make it difficult to take full, deep breaths.

Dealing with Shortness of Breath

Just as there are many causes of shortness of breath, there are many things that you can do to manage this problem.

- *Don't stop what you are doing or hurry up to finish* when you feel short of breath. Instead, *slow down.* If shortness of breath continues, stop for a few minutes. If you are still short of breath, take your medication if it has been prescribed by your doctor. Often shortness of breath is frightening, and this fear can cause two additional problems. First, the hormones that fear can cause the body to release may cause more shortness of breath. Second, fear may cause you to stop your activity and thus never build up the endurance necessary to help your breathing. The basic rule is to take things slowly and in steps.

- *Increase your activity level gradually,* generally not by more than 25 percent each week. Thus, if you are now able to garden comfortably for 20 minutes, next week increase your time by a maximum of 5 minutes. Once you can garden comfortably for 25 minutes, you can again add a few more minutes.

- *Don't smoke.* If you are a smoker, not smoking is easier said than done because most smokers are addicted to smoking and nicotine without realizing it. When you try to quit, the unpleasant symptoms of withdrawal, such as lightheadedness, sleepiness, or headaches, make it very difficult. These symptoms, however, subside in a few weeks but can still leave you with a craving for nicotine. Your doctor can prescribe a nicotine patch or gum to help you through the process of withdrawal. Another alternative is to find ways to distract or occupy yourself until the urge to smoke passes, such as chewing gum, walking around for a few minutes, brushing your teeth, or calling a friend. With time, the urges become less frequent.

In addition to getting over the addiction to nicotine, you may find that the physical motions associated with smoking are hard to change. Try to find something else to keep your hands busy. You may also need to distract yourself or learn to substitute another activity for smoking when you are drinking coffee, finishing meals, reading, or watching television.

For some, it is the fear of failing that keeps them from even trying to quit. Whatever your reasons or difficulties are, however, there are many resources in the community that can help you when you decide to quit, such as the American Cancer Society, the American Heart Association, the American Lung Association, your local community hospital or health maintenance organization, or the health department. Many of these organizations offer courses and/or materials to help you stop on your own or in a group setting.

- *Avoid the smoke of others.* Avoiding "secondary smoke" is as important in managing shortness of breath as stopping smoking. This may sometimes be hard to do because smoking friends may not realize how difficult they are making your life. Your job is to tell them. Explain that their smoke is causing breathing problems for you and you would appreciate it if they would not smoke when you are around. Make your house a No Smoking zone. Ask people to smoke outside.

- *Use your medications and oxygen as prescribed by your doctor.* We are constantly being bombarded by messages that drugs are bad and not to be used. In many cases, this is correct. However, when you have a chronic disease, drugs can be, and often are, life savers. Don't try to skimp, cut down, or go without. Likewise, more is not better, so don't take more than the prescribed amount of medication(s). Drugs, taken as prescribed, can make all the difference. This may mean using medications even when you are not having symptoms. It also means resisting the temptation to take more of the medication if the prescribed amount does not seem to be working. If you have questions about your medications or feel as if they are not working for you, discuss these concerns with your doctor *before* you stop taking the medication or start taking more than has been prescribed. Preventing problems before they start is much better than having to manage the problem later.

- *Drink plenty of fluids* if mucus and secretions are a problem unless your doctor has advised you to restrict your fluid intake. The extra fluids will help to thin the mucus and therefore make it easier to cough up. Using a humidifier may also be helpful.

Pursed-Lip Breathing

Use this technique during exercise or anytime you feel short of breath.

1. *Breathe in through your nose.* This may be easier if you lean forward slightly.

2. *Hold your breath* briefly.

3. *With your lips pursed* as if you were going to whistle, *breathe out slowly* through your lips. Exhaling should take twice as long as inhaling.

4. *Practice this technique for 5 to 10 minutes,* two to four times a day.

Diaphragmatic Breathing

Use this technique to strengthen your breathing muscles.

1. *Lie on your back* with pillows under your head and knees.

2. Place *one hand on your stomach* (at the base of your breastbone) and the *other hand on your upper chest.*

3. *Inhale slowly through your nose,* allowing your stomach to expand outward. Imagine that your lungs are filling with fresh air. The hand on your stomach should move upward, and the hand on your chest should not move.

4. *Breathe out slowly, through pursed lips.* At the same time, use your hand to gently push inward and upward on your abdomen.

5. *Practice this technique for 10 to 15 minutes,* three or four times a day, until it becomes automatic. If you begin to feel a little dizzy, rest.

- *Practice pursed-lip and diaphragmatic breathing.** As mentioned earlier, one of the problems that causes shortness of breath is a deconditioning of the diaphragm and breathing muscles. When this deconditioning occurs, the lungs are not able to empty properly, leaving less room for fresh air. Practiced together, pursed-lip and diaphragmatic breathing can help strengthen and improve the coordination and the efficiency of the breathing muscles as well as decrease the amount of energy needed to breathe. In addition, these two breathing exercises can be used with any

---

*The material on pursed-lip and diaphragmatic breathing was taken from Thomas L. Petty, M.D., Brian Tiep, M.D., and Mary Burns, R.N., B.S., *Essentials of Pulmonary Rehabilitation,* Pulmonary Education and Research Foundation, P.O. Box 1133, Lomita, CA 90717-5133; American Lung Association, *Help Yourself to Better Breathing,* 1989.

of the techniques that use the power of your mind to manage your symptoms (often referred to as cognitive symptom management techniques and described in Chapter 7) or alone, to achieve a state of relaxation.

Diaphragmatic breathing requires a little more practice to master than pursed-lip breathing. Whereas pursed-lip breathing helps to empty the lungs of trapped air and reestablish a normal breathing pattern, diaphragmatic breathing strengthens the breathing muscles. Strengthening these muscles makes them more efficient so less effort is needed to breathe.

Once you feel comfortable with this technique, you may wish to place a light weight on your abdomen. This will further strengthen the muscles you use to inhale. Start with a weight of about 1 pound, like a book or a bag of rice or beans. Gradually increase the weight as your muscle strength improves. After you can breathe easily lying down, you can practice diaphragmatic breathing while sitting, standing, and finally while walking. By mastering this technique while doing other activities, you will be better able to manage your shortness of breath.

Sleeping Problems

Sleep is the time during which the body can concentrate on healing because minimal amounts of energy are required to maintain body functioning when we sleep. When we do not get enough sleep, we can experience a variety of other symptoms, such as fatigue and lack of concentration. This does not mean that fatigue or lack of concentration are always caused by a lack of sleep; remember, the symptoms associated with HIV/AIDS can have many causes. However, if you have noticed a change in your sleep patterns, then the fatigue you are experiencing may, at least in part, be related to your problems with sleep.

Dealing with Sleep Problems

Many people feel powerless to change their sleep problems, but there are many things you can do to help yourself get a good night's sleep. Many of the things that interfere with sleep are quite predictable. To sleep well, you need to (1) have a good, comfortable place to sleep, (2) avoid putting substances in your body that interfere with sleep, (3) get into a sleep routine, and (4) learn to deal with things that might interrupt your sleep. Each of these items is covered below.

Before you even get into bed

- *Get a comfortable bed* that allows for ease of movement and good body support. This usually means a good-quality, firm mattress that supports the spine and does not allow the body to stay in the middle of the bed. A bed board, made of half-inch to three-quarter-inch plywood, can be placed between the mattress and the box spring to increase the firmness. Heated waterbeds or airbeds are helpful for some people because they support weight evenly by conforming to the body's shape. Other people can find them to be very uncomfortable. If you are interested, try one out at a friend's home or a hotel for a few nights to decide if it is right for you.

- *Elevate the head of your bed* on wooden blocks 4 to 6 inches thick to make breathing easier. You can get the same effect by using pillows that elevate your chest, shoulders, and head.

- *Keep the room at a comfortable, warm temperature.*

- *Use a vaporizer* if you live where the air is dry or in cold weather when your heating system will lower the humidity of the air in your house. Warm, moist air often makes breathing easier, leaving you with one less thing to worry about when trying to fall asleep.

- *Make your bedroom a place in which you feel safe and comfortable.* Keep a lamp and telephone by your bed within easy reach.

- *Keep a pair of glasses by the bed* when you go to sleep if you are nearsighted and wear glasses or contact lenses. This way, in case you need to get up in the middle of the night, you can easily put on your glasses and see where you are going!

Things to avoid before bedtime

- *Avoid eating before bedtime.* Although you may feel sleepy after eating a big meal, eating is no way to help you fall asleep and get a good night's sleep. Sleep is supposed to allow your body time to rest and recover, but when you eat, your body is kept busy with digestion; taking valuable time away from this healing process. Since going to sleep feeling hungry may also keep you awake, try drinking a glass of warm milk.

- *Avoid alcohol.* Contrary to the popular belief that alcohol will help you to sleep better because it makes you feel more relaxed, alcohol actually disrupts your sleep cycle. Alcohol before bedtime can lead to shallow and fragmented sleep, as well as frequent awakenings throughout the night.

- *Avoid caffeine late in the day.* Because caffeine is a stimulant, it can keep you awake. In addition to coffee, caffeine is also found in some types of teas, colas and other sodas, and chocolate.

- *Avoid eating foods with MSG (monosodium glutamate) late in the day.* Although Chinese foods often have been singled out as containing MSG, many other types of food, especially prepackaged foods, may contain this food additive. Before purchasing a prepackaged meal, be sure to read the ingredient label to make sure the food does not contain monosodium glutamate.

- *Don't smoke to help you sleep.* The nicotine contained in cigarettes is a stimulant. And aside from the fact that smoking itself can cause complications and a worsening of lung problems, falling asleep with a lit cigarette can be a fire hazard.

- *Avoid diet pills.* Diet pills often contain stimulants that may interfere with falling asleep as well as staying asleep.

- *Avoid sleeping pills.* Although the name *sleeping pills* sounds like the perfect solution for sleep problems, they tend to become less effective over time. Also, many sleeping pills have a rebound effect—that is, if you stop taking them, it is more difficult to get to sleep. Thus, as they become less effective, you have even more problems than you had when you first started taking the sleeping pills. It is best to avoid using sleeping pills if at all possible.

Developing a routine

- *Set up a regular rest and sleep pattern.* Go to bed at the same time every night and get up at the same time every morning. If you wish to take a nap, take one in the afternoon, but do not take a nap after dinner. Stay awake until you are ready to go to bed.

- *Reset your sleep clock if your sleep pattern is way off the norm* (for example, if you go to bed at 4:00 A.M. and sleep until noon). To do so, try going to bed one hour earlier or later each day until you reach the hour you want to go to bed. This method may seem strange, but it seems to be the best way to reset your sleep clock.

- *Exercise at regular times each day.* Not only will the exercise help you have better quality sleep, exercising at the same time every day will also help to set a regular pattern for your day.

- *Get out in the sun every afternoon,* even if it is only for 15 or 20 minutes. The sun is necessary to keep your "body clock" correctly set.

- Get used to doing the *same things every night before going to bed*. This can be anything from watching the news, to reading a chapter of a book, to taking a warm bath. By developing and sticking to a getting-ready-for-bed routine, you will be telling your body that it's time to start winding down and relax.

But I can't fall (back) asleep

- *Only use your bed and your bedroom for sleeping or for sex*. If you find that you get into bed and you can't fall asleep, get out of bed and go into another room until you begin to feel sleepy again.
- *Don't keep a TV set in the bedroom*. Many people have a TV set in their bedroom, thinking that it helps them fall asleep. It doesn't. It actually keeps the mind racing and interferes with sleep. You might think, "But I always fall asleep with the TV on!" But do you ever fall asleep *early* with it on? Not likely. Probably it's sometime during the late show!
- *Refocus your mind away from worries*. Many people can get to sleep without a problem but then wake up and have the "early morning worries," in which they can't turn off their mind. Then they get more worried because they cannot go back to sleep once they have awakened. Keeping your mind fully occupied will ward off the worries and help you get back to sleep. For example, try quieting your mind by counting backward from 100 by threes, naming a flower for every letter of the alphabet, or some other type of distraction.
- *Don't worry about not getting enough sleep*. If your body needs sleep, you will sleep. Also, remember that people tend to need less sleep as they get older.

Stress

Stress is a common problem for everyone. But what *is* stress? In the 1950s, physiologist Hans Selye described stress as "the nonspecific response of the body to any demand made upon it." Others have expanded this definition to explain that the body adapts to demands, whether pleasant or unpleasant.

How Does Your Body Respond to Stress?

Your body is used to functioning at a certain level. When there is a need to change this level, your body must adjust physiologically to meet the demand.

Your body reacts by preparing itself to take an action: your heart rate increases, your blood pressure rises, your neck and shoulder muscles tense, your breathing becomes more rapid, your digestion slows, your mouth becomes dry, and you may begin sweating. These are typical signals of stress.

What causes stress responses?

To take an action, your muscles need a supply of oxygen and energy. Your rate of breathing increases in an effort to inhale as much oxygen as possible and to get rid of as much carbon dioxide as possible. Your heart rate increases to deliver the oxygen and nutrients to the muscles. Furthermore, physiological processes that are not immediately necessary, such as the digestion of food and the body's natural immune responses, are slowed.

How long will stress responses last?

In general, stress responses are present only until the stressful event passes. Your body then returns to its normal level of functioning. Sometimes, though, your body does not return to its former comfortable level. If the stress is present for any length of time, your body begins adapting to this stress. This adaptation can contribute to the development of health problems such as hypertension (high blood pressure), shortness of breath, or painful joints.

Common Types of Stressors

Regardless of the type of stressor (the initiator of a stress response), the changes in the body are the same. Stressors, however, are not completely independent of one another. In fact, one stressor can often lead to other types of stressors or even magnify existing stressors. Several stressors can also occur simultaneously. This is much the same as the vicious cycle of deconditioning and helplessness described in Chapter 1.

Some of the more common sources and types of stress include:

- *Physical stressors.* Physical stressors can range from something as pleasant as going out dancing, to grocery shopping, to something unpleasant, like the physical symptoms of your HIV/AIDS. The one thing that these three stressors have in common is that they all increase your body's demand for energy. If your body is not prepared to deal with this demand, the results may be sore muscles, fatigue, and a worsening of some disease symptoms.

- *Mental and emotional stressors.* Mental and emotional stressors can range from pleasant to uncomfortable. The joys you experience seeing your sister get married or meeting new friends induce the same stress response in the body as feeling frustrated or down because of your illness. Although it seems strange that this is true, the difference comes in the way the stress is perceived by your brain.

- *Environmental stressors.* Environmental stressors can also be good or bad. They may be as varied as a sunny day, uneven sidewalks that make it difficult to walk, loud noises, bad weather, or secondhand smoke.

Isn't "Good Stress" a Contradiction?

As we mentioned earlier, some types of stress can be good. A job promotion, a wedding, a vacation, a new friendship, or a new baby makes you feel good but still causes the same physiological changes in your body. Another example of a "good stressor" is exercise.

When you exercise or do any type of physical activity, a demand is placed on the body. The heart has to work harder to deliver blood to the muscles, the lungs are working harder, and you breathe more rapidly to keep up with your muscles' demand for oxygen. Meanwhile, your muscles are working hard to keep up with the signals from your brain that are telling them to keep moving. As you maintain an exercise program for several weeks, you will begin to notice a change: what once seemed virtually impossible is now relatively simple. Your body has adapted to this stress. In addition, there is less strain on your heart, lungs, and other muscles to do this 5 minutes of activity. They've become more efficient, and you have become more fit.

Recognizing When You Feel Stressed

In reality, you have a certain need for stress—it helps your life run more efficiently. As long as you don't go past your breaking point, stress is helpful. Some days you can tolerate more stress than others. But sometimes, if you are not aware of the different types of stress you are experiencing, you can go beyond your breaking point and feel like your life is completely out of control. Often it is difficult to recognize when you are under too much stress.

The warning signs of stress include:

- biting your nails, pulling your hair, or other repetitive habits
- grinding your teeth, clenching your jaw
- tension in your head, neck, or shoulders (which can cause headaches)
- feelings of anxiousness, nervousness, helplessness, or irritability

Sometimes you can catch yourself in these stress responses. If you do, take a few minutes to think about what it is that is making you feel tense. Take a few deep breaths and try to relax. Some methods for using your mind to help you relax are presented in Chapter 7.

Dealing with Stress

Stress can't be "cured," because it's part and parcel of everyday life. But you can learn to deal with the bad effects of stress. Two ways of coping with stress are: (1) *avoiding* stressful situations and (2) *managing* stressful situations.

Avoiding Stressful Situations

Some situations are immediately identifiable as being stressful—for example, being stuck in traffic, going on a trip, or preparing a meal. First, *look, as objectively as possible, at what it is about the particular situation that is stressful.* Is it that you hate to be late? Are trips stressful because of the uncertainty involved with your destination? Does meal preparation involve too many steps that demand too much energy?

Once you have decided on what specifically is stressful about a situation, you can *begin looking for possible ways to avoid the aspects of the situation that are creating stress for you.* Can you leave earlier? Can you let someone else drive? Can you call someone at your destination site and ask about wheelchair access, local mass transit, and so on? Can you prepare food in the morning? Can you take a short nap in the early afternoon? After you have identified some possible solutions, *select one* to try the next time you are in this situation. Don't forget to *evaluate the results.* (This is the problem-solving approach we discussed in Chapter 2.)

Managing the Stress

Although you can successfully manage some types of stress by avoiding the stressful parts of the situation, many other types of stress seem to sneak up on you when you don't expect them. Dealing with this type of stress also involves the problem-solving approach.

If you know that certain situations will be stressful, *develop ways to deal with them before they happen.* Try to *rehearse*, in your mind, what you will do when the situation arises, so you will be ready. Inherent in this approach is listening to your body for signals that the tension and stress are building. The better you become at listening and understanding your body's signals, the better you'll become at managing your stress and stressful situations.

Certain chemicals such as nicotine, alcohol, and caffeine, can also increase stress. Although you may smoke a cigarette, drink a glass of wine, or drink a cup of coffee to soothe your tension, these substances, in fact, actually increase the stress response in your body. Eliminating these stressors can leave you feeling calmer.

Chapter 5, "Using Your Mind to Manage Symptoms," discusses mental techniques, such as self-talk, progressive muscle relaxation, guided imagery, and visualization, that may also be useful to you in stressful situations. Additional ways to deal with stress, such as getting enough sleep, exercising, and eating well, are discussed in other chapters of this book. See Chapters 5, 6, and 7.

In summary, stress, like every other symptom, has many causes and, therefore, has more than one way to be managed. It is up to you to examine the problem and try those solutions that meet your needs and lifestyle.

Taking actions to physically deal with your symptoms is necessary in coping with your illness on a day-to-day basis. But sometimes, this just doesn't seem to be enough. There are times during the day when you may wish to escape from your surroundings and just have "your time"—a time that allows you to clear your mind, to gain a fresh perspective. The following chapter will show you different ways to complement your physical symptom management with *cognitive techniques*—techniques in which you use your mind to help reduce and even prevent some of the symptoms you may experience.

Suggested Reading

Lewinsohn, Peter, with Ricardo Munoz, Mary Youngren, and Antoinette Zeiss. *Control Your Depression*. New York: Prentice Hall, 1987.

5

Using Your Mind
to Manage Symptoms

All of us, at one time or another, have experienced the power of the mind and its effect on the body. For example, when we are embarrassed, we feel flushed and our faces blush. If we think about sucking on a lemon, our mouths pucker and we salivate. Thoughts and feelings, pleasant and unpleasant, can affect our breathing and our heart rate. In fact, some people with breathing problems get short of breath just thinking about exercising.

These simple examples prove the power of the mind and its ability to affect the body. Through training and practice, you can learn to use your mind to relax your body, to reduce stress and anxiety, and to decrease discomfort or unpleasantness caused by physical and emotional symptoms. Your mind can effectively help you to relieve symptoms common to many different diseases. The mind is particularly helpful in managing pain and shortness of breath, and may even help you depend less on drugs.

This chapter describes several techniques, called *cognitive techniques*, that use the power of your mind to help you manage your disease symptoms. All of these techniques are designed for you to use at home. These same techniques are the basis of biofeedback training, a technique whereby one's ability to make changes in the body (that is, relax muscles, raise hand temperature, or slow a heart rate) is monitored by sensitive instruments whose sound provides feedback on one's success.

There are many different ways to try to use the powerful influence the mind has over the body. *Muscle relaxation* is one of the most important for chronic pain control, because so much chronic pain is intensified by muscle tension and spasm. Relaxation through *guided imagery* and *visualization* can lead to a meditation-like state in which many body processes are affected. *Self-talk* is based on the idea that how we think about a task affects how we experience it. For example, an athlete who is convinced she can't make a jump is unlikely to make it; on the other hand, knowing in your mind you can make something happen may be the key to success. Finally, *distraction, dissociation,* and *relabeling* are techniques that can help you to use the brain to lessen uncomfortable feelings. All of these techniques are discussed below.

Relaxation Techniques

Although you may have heard and read about relaxation, you may still be confused as to what it is, what its benefits are, and how to do it. Relaxation is not a cure-all, but neither is it a hoax or a silly mind game. Rather, like other treatment methods, it has specific guidelines and specific uses. Some techniques are used only to achieve muscle relaxation; others are aimed at reducing anxiety and emotional arousal or at diverting attention, all of which aid in symptom management.

The term *relaxation* means different things to different people: We can all identify ways we relax. For example, we may walk, watch TV, play golf, cook, or garden. These methods of relaxing, however, are different from the techniques discussed here because they include some form of physical activity that requires your mind's attention. Relaxation techniques are also different from napping in that they require us to use our minds actively to help our bodies achieve a relaxed state. *The goal of relaxation is to turn off the outside world so the mind and body are at rest.* This state allows you to reduce the tension that increases the intensity of symptoms. When you have become adept at using

---

Guidelines for Using Relaxation Techniques

- *Pick a quiet place and time* during the day when you will not be disturbed for at least 15–20 minutes.
- *Try to practice the technique twice daily,* but not less than 4 times a week.
- *Don't expect miracles.* Some of these techniques take time to acquire the skill and sometimes 3 to 4 weeks of practice before you really start to notice benefits.
- *Relaxation should be helpful.* At worst, you may find it boring, but if it is an unpleasant experience or makes you more nervous or anxious, then you might do better with other symptom management techniques.

---

the relaxation techniques described below, you will find that your relaxation sessions leave you with an overall feeling of peace and well-being, as well as a lessening of your physical symptoms.

Muscle Relaxation

Muscle relaxation is one of the most commonly used cognitive techniques for symptom management. It is popular because it makes sense to us. If we are told that physical stress or muscular tension intensifies our pain, shortness of breath, or emotional distress, we are motivated to learn how to recognize this tension and release it. In addition, muscle relaxation is easy to learn and to recall for practice in different situations. It is one technique in which we can recognize some immediate results, such as the positive sensations of reduced pain, stress, or muscle tension and calm, normal breathing. Muscle relaxation

Progressive Muscle Relaxation Exercise

This exercise guides you through the major muscle groups, asking you to first *tense*, and then to *relax*, those muscles. If you have pain in a particular area today, tense those muscles only gently or not at all and focus on relaxing them.

1. Make yourself as comfortable as possible. Loosen any clothing that feels tight. Uncross your legs and ankles. Allow your body to feel supported by the surface on which you are sitting or lying.

2. Close your eyes. Take a deep breath, filling your chest and breathing all the way down to the abdomen. Hold . . . Breathe out through pursed lips and as you breathe out, let as much tension as possible flow out with your breath. Let all your muscles feel heavy and let your whole body just sink into the surface beneath you . . . Good.

3. Become aware of the muscles in your *feet and calves*. Pull your toes back up toward your knees. Notice the tension in your feet and calves. Release and relax. Notice the discomfort leaving as relief and warmth replace it. That's it.

4. Now tighten the muscles of your *thighs and buttocks*. Hold and feel the tension. Let go and allow the muscles to relax. The relaxed muscles feel heavy and supported by the surface upon which you are sitting or lying.

5. Tense the muscles in your *abdomen and chest*. Notice a tendency to hold your breath as you tense. Relax, and notice that it is natural to want to take a deep breath to relieve the tension in this area. Take a deep breath

is not likely to fail because of distractions caused by symptoms or thoughts. It is a useful strategy to reduce pain, muscular tension, and stress while helping to control shortness of breath and to achieve a more restful sleep.

The following are two examples of muscle relaxation techniques. Try both techniques and choose the one that works best for you. Then tape record the script for that routine. Although recording the script is not necessary, it is sometimes helpful if you find it hard to concentrate. Also, you won't be distracted by having to refer to the book when you are trying to relax.

Progressive Muscle Relaxation

Many years ago, a physiologist named Edmund Jacobson discovered that in order to relax, one must know how it feels to be tense, as well as relaxed. He believed that if one learned to recognize tension, then one could learn to let it go and relax. He designed a simple exercise to assist with this learning process.

(continued)

now, breathing all the way down to the abdomen. As you breathe out, allow all the tension to flow out with your breath.

6. Now, stretching your fingers out straight, tense your fingers and tighten your *arm muscles*. Relax. Feel the tension flowing out as the circulation returns.

7. Press your shoulder blades together, tightening the muscles in your *shoulders and neck*. This is a place where many people carry a lot of tension. Hold . . . Now, let go. Notice how the muscles feel warmer and more alive.

8. Tighten all the muscles of your *face and head*. Notice the tension, especially around your eyes and in your jaw. Now relax, allowing your jaw to become slack and your mouth to remain slightly open . . . That's right. Note the difference.

9. Now take another deep breath, breathing all the way down to the abdomen. And, as you breathe out, allow your body to sink heavily into the surface beneath you, becoming even more deeply relaxed. Good.

10. Enjoy this comfortable feeling of relaxation . . . Remember it. With practice, you will become skilled at recognizing muscle tension and releasing it . . .

11. Prepare to come back into the here and now. Take three deep breaths. When you're ready, open your eyes.

To relax muscles you need to know how to scan your body, recognize where you are holding tension, and release that tension. The first step is to become familiar with the difference between the feeling of *tension* and the feeling of *relaxation*. The brief progressive muscle relaxation exercise on pages 72–73 will allow you to compare those feelings and, with practice, spot and release tension anywhere in your body.

As Jacobson emphasizes in the exercise, the purpose of voluntarily tensing the muscles is to learn to recognize and locate tension in your body. You will then become aware of tension and use this same procedure of letting go. *Once you learn the technique it will no longer be necessary to tense voluntarily; just locate the existing tension and let it go.*

For some people with a lot of pain, particularly in the joints, the Jacobson progressive muscle relaxation technique may not be appropriate. If it causes any pain, the pain may distract you from the relaxation. If this is the case, the relaxation response technique may work better for you.

The Relaxation Response

In the early 1970s a physician named Herbert Benson studied extensively what he calls the *relaxation response*. According to Benson, our bodies have several natural states. One is the fight-or-flight response experienced when we are faced with a great danger. In the fight-or-flight response, the body becomes quite tense, followed by its natural tendency to relax. However, as our lives become more and more hectic, our bodies tend to stay in an extended or constant state of tension, and we find it more and more difficult to relax.

The relaxation response exercise on the opposite page is designed to elicit the natural relaxation response of your body. The technique is very much like meditation, for it is based on the principles of meditation.

Imagery

Although the two techniques we have just explored are specifically focused on muscle relaxation, reduction of muscle tension is the most common benefit of all relaxation techniques. You will gain additional emotional and mental benefits from relaxation techniques such as *guided imagery* and *visualization*, which are aimed at helping you reduce fear and anxiety and at refocusing your attention away from the discomfort of symptoms.

The Relaxation Response

To practice the relaxation response you need the following basic elements:

- *A quiet environment.* Turn off all external distractions and internal physical or emotional stimuli.

- *A mental device—that is, an object to dwell upon.* For example, you can repeat a word or sound like the word *one*; gaze at a symbol like a candle or flower; or concentrate on a feeling, such as peace.

- *A passive attitude.* This is the most essential element. You will need to empty all thoughts and distractions from your mind. Thoughts, images, and feelings may drift into awareness, but don't concentrate on them. Just allow them to pass on.

- *A comfortable position.* You should be comfortable enough to remain in the same position for 20 minutes.

You are now ready to elicit the relaxation response:

1. *Sit quietly* in a comfortable position.

2. *Close your eyes.*

3. *Relax all your muscles*, releasing tension in your feet and progressing up to your face. The muscle relaxation skills from the previous section may help you to do this. Keep your muscles relaxed.

4. *Breathe in through your nose.* Become aware of your breathing. As you breathe out through your mouth, *say the word* one *silently to yourself.* Try to *empty all thoughts* from your mind; concentrate on *one.* As you get better at using this technique, you can concentrate on a symbol or a feeling instead, but it's important to be focused—that is, don't try to concentrate on three things all at once.

5. *Continue* this process for 10–20 minutes. You may open your eyes to check the time, but do not use an alarm. When you finish, sit quietly for several minutes, at first with your eyes closed. Do not stand up for a few minutes.

6. Do not worry about whether you are successful in achieving a deep level of relaxation. *Maintain a passive attitude* and let relaxation occur at its own pace. When distracting thoughts occur, ignore them by not dwelling upon them, and return to repeating the word *one.*

7. *Practice* this technique once or twice daily, but ideally not within 2 hours after any meal. Digestive processes can interfere with relaxation responses.

Guided Imagery

The guided imagery relaxation technique is like a guided daydream. It allows you to divert your attention, refocusing your mind away from your symptoms and transporting you to another time and place. It also has the added dimension of helping you to achieve deep relaxation by picturing yourself in a peaceful environment. The two guided imagery scripts presented here can help take you on this mental stroll.

A WALK IN THE COUNTRY   *Guided Imagery*

- Make yourself as comfortable as possible, sitting or lying down. Loosen any constricting clothing. Uncross your arms, legs, and ankles. Allow your body to feel supported by the surface on which you are sitting or lying.
- Close your eyes.
- Take a deep breath, in through your nose, breathing all the way down to the abdomen. Hold . . . Breathe out slowly through slightly pursed lips and as you do, relax your whole body, allowing all your muscles to feel limp and heavy . . . Good.
- Scan your body for any muscle tension, starting with your head and going all the way down to your toes.
- Release any tension in your face, head, and neck by letting your jaw become slack and your head feel heavy on your shoulders. Allow your shoulders to drop heavily. Take a deep breath and relax your chest and abdomen. Allow your arms and legs to feel heavy and to sink into the surface beneath you.
- Now take a deep breath and become aware of any remaining tension in your body. As you breathe out, allow all the muscles of your body to sink heavily into the surface beneath you, becoming even more deeply relaxed . . . Good.
- Imagine yourself walking along an old country road . . . the sun is warm on your back . . . the birds are singing . . . the air is calm and fragrant.
- As you progress down the road, you come across an old gate . . . The gate creaks as you open it and go through.
- You find yourself in an overgrown garden, flowers growing where they have

---

There are several ways in which you can use the following guided imagery scripts:

- You can read the script over several times to familiarize yourself with it. Then sit or lie down in a quiet place and try to reconstruct the scene in your mind. Each script should take 10–15 minutes to complete.
- You can have a family member or friend read you the script slowly, pausing for 5–10 seconds wherever there is a series of dots (. . .).
- You can make a tape of the script and play it to yourself whenever convenient.

(continued)

seeded themselves, vines climbing over a fallen tree, green grass, shade trees.

- Breathe deeply, smelling the flowers . . . listen to the birds and insects . . . feel the gentle breeze, warm against your skin.
- As you walk leisurely up a gentle slope behind the garden, you come to a wooded area where the trees become denser and the sun is filtered through the leaves. The air feels mild and a bit cooler. You become aware of the sound and fragrance of a nearby brook. You breathe deeply of the cool and fragrant air several times, and with each breath you feel more refreshed.
- Soon you come upon the brook. It is clear and clean as it tumbles over the rocks and some fallen logs. You follow the path along the brook for a ways. The path takes you out into a sunlit clearing where you discover a small and picturesque waterfall . . . There is a rainbow in the mist . . .
- You find a comfortable place to sit for a while, a perfect niche where you can feel completely relaxed.
- You feel good as you allow yourself to just enjoy the warmth and solitude of this peaceful place.
- It is now time to return. You walk back down the path, through the cool and fragrant trees, out into the sun-drenched overgrown garden . . . one last smell of the flowers, and out the creaky gate . . .
- You leave this secret retreat for now and return down the country road. However, you know that you may visit this special place whenever you wish.
- When you are ready, take three deep breaths and open your eyes whenever you wish.

| **A HAPPY TIME** | **Guided Imagery** |

- Before imagining or listening to this scene, close your eyes and take three deep breaths . . . breathe slowly and easily, in through your nose and out through your mouth . . .

- Now picture a happy, pleasant time, a time when you have little or no problems or worries about your health . . .

- Fill in the details of this time . . . look at the surroundings . . . are they indoors? . . . outdoors? . . . who is there? . . . what are you doing? . . . listen to the noises . . . even those in the background . . . are there any pleasant smells? . . . feel the temperature . . . now, just enjoy your surroundings . . . you are happy . . . your body feels good . . . enjoy your surroundings . . . fix this feeling in your mind . . . you can return any time you wish by just picturing this happy time . . .

- When you are ready, take three deep breaths . . . with each breath say the word *relax* . . . imagine the word written in warm sand . . . now open your eyes . . . remain quiet for a few moments before slowly returning to your activities.

Visualization

Visualization, also referred to as *vivid imagery*, is similar to guided imagery. It is another way of using the imagination to picture yourself any way you want, doing things you want to do. You can practice visualization in different ways and for longer, as well as brief, periods. You can also use this relaxation technique while you are engaged in other activities.

One way to use visualization is to recall pleasant scenes from your past or create new scenes in your mind. It allows you to create more of your own images than the guided imagery technique does. For example, try to remember every detail of a special holiday or party that made you happy. Who was there? What happened? What did you talk about? You can do the same sort of thing by remembering a vacation. In fact, visualization can also be used to plan the details of some future event. In this case, try to fill in the details of a pleasant fantasy. For example, how would you spend a million dollars? What would be your ideal romantic encounter? What would your ideal home or garden look like? Where would you go and what would you do on your dream vacation?

Another form of visualization involves imagining symbols that represent the discomfort of pain felt in different parts of your body. For example, a painful joint might be red, or a tight chest might have a constricting band around it. After forming these images, you then try to change them. The red color might fade until there is no more color, or the constricting band might stretch and stretch until it falls off. Visualization is a useful technique to help you set and accomplish your personal goals (see Chapter 2). After you write your weekly contract, take a few minutes to imagine yourself taking a walk, doing your exercises, or taking your medications. Here you are mentally rehearsing the steps you need to take in order to achieve your contract successfully. Studies have shown that this technique can help people cope better with stressful situations, master skills, and accomplish personal goals. In fact, those people who have become skilled at visualization find they can actually decrease some of the discomfort and distress associated with symptoms by changing unpleasant images to pleasant ones.

All the relaxation techniques mentioned above can be used in conjunction with pursed-lip breathing and diaphragmatic breathing. These two breathing methods, described in Chapter 4, can help you achieve a more relaxed state and keep your mind off the potential for shortness of breath.

Other Cognitive Strategies

Other cognitive strategies, such as *meditation* and *reflection* take a different approach to managing symptoms. These techniques all involve retraining your patterns of thinking so that chronic pains seem less intense, less limiting, or less important.

Self-Talk—"I Know I Can"

All of us talk to ourselves all the time. For example, when waking up in the morning, we think, "I really don't want to get out of bed. I'm tired and don't want to go to work today." Or, at the end of an enjoyable evening, we think, "Gee, that was fun. I should get out more often." These things we think or say to ourselves are called "self-talk."

All of our self-talk is learned from others and becomes a part of us as we grow up. It comes in many forms, mostly negative. Negative self-statements are usually in the form of: "I just can't do . . . ," "If only I could or didn't . . . ," "I just don't have the energy. . . ." This type of self-talk represents the doubts and fears we have about ourselves in general and about our abilities to deal with a disease and its symptoms in particular. Unfortunately, negative self-talk can have the effect of worsening symptoms like pain, depression, and fatigue.

Because what we learn in life influences our beliefs, attitudes, feelings, and actions, what we say to ourselves plays a major role in determining our success or failure in becoming good self-managers. Learning to make self-talk work *for* you instead of *against* you, by changing those negative statements to positive ones, will help you manage your symptoms more effectively. This change, as with any habit, requires practice.

To change negative self-talk to positive:

1. *Listen carefully to what you say* to *or* about *yourself*, both out loud and silently. Then write down all the negative self-talk statements. Pay special attention to the things you say during times that are particularly difficult for you. For example, what do you say to yourself when getting up in the morning with pain, while doing those exercises you don't really like, or at those times when you are feeling blue?

2. *Work on* changing *each negative statement you identified to a positive one*, and write these down. Positive statements should reflect the better you and your decision to be in control. For example, the negative statements—such as, "I don't want to get up," "I'm too tired and I hurt," "I can't do the things I like anymore so why bother," or "I'm good for nothing,"—become positive messages—such as "I have the energy to get up and do the things I enjoy," "I know I can do anything I believe I can," "People like me and I feel good about myself," or "Other people need and depend on me. I'm worthwhile."

3. *Read and rehearse these positive statements*, mentally or with another person. It is this conscious repetition or memorization of positive self-talk that will help you replace those old, habitual negative statements.

4. *Practice these new statements in real situations.* This practice, along with time and patience, will help your new patterns of thinking become automatic.

Once established, positive self-talk can be one of the most powerful tools you can add to your self-management program, helping you to manage symptoms as well as to master the other skills discussed in this book.

Distraction

Because our minds have trouble focusing on more than one thing at a time, you can lessen the intensity of your symptoms by training your mind to focus attention on something other than your body and its sensations. This technique, called *distraction* or *attention refocusing*, is particularly helpful if you feel your symptoms are overwhelming or worry that every bodily sensation might indicate a new or worsening symptom or health problem. It is important to mention that with distraction you are not ignoring the symptoms, but choosing not to dwell on them.

Distraction works best for short activities or episodes in which symptoms may be anticipated, as in the following examples:

- *Make plans for exactly what you will do after the unpleasant activity passes.* For example, if climbing stairs is uncomfortable or painful, think about what you need to do once you get to the top. If you have trouble falling asleep, try making plans for some future event, being as detailed as possible.

- *Try to think of a person's name, a bird, a flower, and so on, for every letter of the alphabet.* If you get stuck on one letter, go on to the next. (These are good distractions for pain as well as for sleep problems.)

- *Try counting backward* from 1,000 or 100 by threes (for example, 100, 97, 94, . . .).

- *To get through unpleasant daily chores* (such as sweeping, mopping, or vacuuming), *imagine your floor as a map of a country or continent.* Try naming all the states, provinces, or countries, moving east to west or north to south. If geography does not appeal to you, imagine your favorite store and where each department is located.

- *Try to remember words to favorite songs or the events in an old story.* There are, of course, a million variations to these examples, all of which help you to refocus attention away from your problem.

So far we have discussed short-term distraction strategies in which you refocus your mind *internally*, away from your symptoms to thoughts of something more pleasant. There is another kind of distraction, the distraction of action, that works well for long-term projects or symptoms that tend to last longer, such as depression and some forms of chronic pain. In this type of distraction, the mind is not focused internally, but rather *externally*, on some type of activity. If you are slightly depressed or have continuous unpleasant symptoms, find an activity that interests you and you will find yourself distracted from the problem. This activity can be almost anything from gardening, to cooking, to reading, to going to a movie, or even doing volunteer work. One of the marks of a successful self-manager is that he or she has a variety of interests and always seems to be doing something.

Dissociation

Dissociation is a technique that goes further than distraction and that is often difficult to master. It involves mentally separating yourself from the physical sensations or symptoms of your body. It is especially effective when physical symptoms, such as pain, are so severe that it is difficult or impossible to distract yourself.

To use dissociation, picture the painful or uncomfortable part of your body as separate from the rest of your body. Imagine that this body part is completely insensitive and therefore does not feel anything. It does not belong to you; it is completely separate from you. You cannot feel anything that happens to it. Whatever happens to this part does not affect you at all. You can even imagine that you have floated away from your body and are looking at it from across the room.

Relabeling

Any symptom can be thought of as a combination of sensations you feel in your body. Relabeling is a technique that you can use to deal with symptoms like pain, fatigue, and depression by thinking about the sensations that make up the symptom. Relabeling is the opposite of distraction or attention refocusing because, rather than thinking of something else, you will think about the problem. In fact, you will do more than that. You will try to analyze it. For example, if you have "pain," are the sensations sharp? Dull? Hot? Cold? If you are having "depression," what are these sensations like? Are they mild or intense, sad or angry? If you are "fatigued," is it weariness or extreme exhaustion? Ask yourself exactly what you are feeling. Now, concentrate on your pulse, breathing, muscle tension, or any thoughts and feelings you may have, but don't think of these sensations as "pain," "depression," or "fatigue." Try thinking of them differently. For example, the "pain" sensations may become mere dullness, the negative feelings of "depression" may become numbness, and "fatigue" sensations may become sleepiness and an opportunity to rest. As the way you think about the sensation changes, the level of the sensation may decrease, increase, or level off. Just go along with it and see if you can change (or *relabel*) the way you think about the sensation.

With practice, this technique can help you lessen the intensity of symptoms, not by diverting your attention as distraction does, but by training your mind to change the way it thinks about, or labels, those symptoms.

Prayer, Meditation, or Reflection

Over the years, many people with chronic illness have told us that prayer, meditation, or reflection have been helpful in managing both the physical and emotional symptoms of their disease. For some, these practices are forms of relaxation that help reduce tension and anxiety. For others, these activities of the mind may be a method of distraction or dissociation, by which they refocus their attention or separate themselves from their symptoms. Regardless of the rationale, prayer, meditation, or reflection are important parts of many people's self-management programs and remain the oldest of all symptom management techniques.

As we mentioned earlier in this book, symptoms, their causes, and the ways they interact to affect your daily life can become a tangled mesh of threads. Identifying your symptoms and their causes begins the untangling process. In the last three chapters we have given you many techniques for identifying, understanding, and managing your symptoms. In concluding this section, we ask you to remember the four basic principles of symptom self-management given in the box below.

Principles of Symptom Self-Management

- *Symptoms have many causes.* Thus, there are many ways to manage most symptoms. Understanding the nature and varied causes of your symptoms and how these interact will help you to better manage your symptoms.

- *Not all management techniques will work for everyone.* It is up to you to experiment and find out what works best for you. Be flexible. This includes trying different techniques and monitoring the results to determine which technique is most helpful for which symptom(s) and under what circumstances.

- *Give yourself several weeks to practice a new symptom management technique* before you decide for sure whether it is working for you. Remember that learning a new skill and gaining control of the situation takes time.

- *Don't give up, even if you feel you are not accomplishing anything.* As is the case with exercise and other acquired skills, using your mind to manage your illness requires both practice and time before you notice the benefits. Be patient and keep on trying!

Suggested Reading

Burns, David D. *Feeling Good: The New Mood Therapy*. New York: Avon Books, 1992.

Davis, Martha, Elizabeth Robbins Eshelman, and Matthew McKay. *The Relaxation and Stress Reduction Workbook*. 2nd ed. Oakland, Calif.: New Harbinger Publications, 1982.

Ornstein, Robert, and David Sobel. *Healthy Pleasures*. Reading, Mass.: Addison-Wesley, 1989.

Managing Exercise and Diet

6

Exercising for Fun and Fitness

The spirit of exercise and fitness is everywhere. Well, almost every-where. Some people with HIV/AIDS often find it difficult to enjoy an active lifestyle. When you want to exercise but aren't sure what to do, physical and emotional limitations from HIV/AIDS can be powerful forces to overcome. Until recently, many people with HIV/AIDS have avoided exercise, thinking that exercising for fun and fitness was only for others. In addition, medical advisors have previously warned people with chronic health problems to avoid strenuous activity. If such people wanted to exercise, they were usually prescribed only very light stretching or range-of-motion exercises. Although these exercises are still important parts of HIV/AIDS management, they needn't be the only exercise for most people.

New research has changed the way we think about exercise and chronic illnesses. Thanks to the knowledge gained from people with chronic illnesses who have worked with health professionals, *we can now advise exercise for fun and fitness.* Exercising regularly lessens fatigue, builds stronger muscles and bones, increases flexibility, produces stamina, and improves general health and the sense of well-being . . . all important in the management of chronic health problems. Research shows that people with chronic health problems as diverse as osteoarthritis, heart disease, chronic lung diseases, and stroke have improved fitness by walking, bicycling, or aquatic exercise. After two or three months, many exercisers also report less pain, less shortness of breath, less anxiety, and less depression. There's no reason that HIV/AIDS should be any different.

Traditional medical care of chronic illness has been based on helping people mainly when their illness worsened and has involved a recommendation to decrease physical activity and increase medical therapy. Unfortunately, long periods of inactivity in anyone can lead to weakness, stiffness, fatigue, poor appetite, constipation, high blood pressure, muscle loss, osteoporosis, and increased sensitivity to pain, anxiety, and depression. These same inactivity-related problems are caused by the illness itself, so it can be difficult to tell whether it is the illness, inactivity, or a combination of the two that is responsible for these problems.

In this chapter, you will learn how to improve your fitness and make wise exercise choices. This advice is not intended to take the place of specific therapeutic recommendations from your doctor or physical therapist. If you've had an exercise plan prescribed for you that differs from the suggestions here, take this book to your doctor or physical therapist and ask what he or she thinks about this program.

Regular exercise benefits many people with chronic health problems, improving levels of strength, energy, and self-confidence, and lessening anxiety and depression. In addition, strong muscles can help people with neuropathy (pain due to decreased nerve function) by improving stability and absorbing shock. Many people with neuropathy can walk farther without leg pain after a regular exercise program. Regular exercise also helps nourish joints and keep cartilage and bone healthy. Regular exercise has been shown to help people with chronic lung problems improve endurance and reduce shortness of breath (and trips to the emergency room!). Finally, regular exercise is usually an essential component of maintaining a healthy weight.

The good news is that it doesn't take hours of painful, sweat-soaked exercise to achieve most of these health benefits. Even short periods of gentle physical activity can significantly improve fitness, reduce health risks, and boost your mood.

Exercise reconditions your body, helping to restore function previously lost to disuse and illness. This will help you improve your health, feel better, and manage your illness better. Feeling more in control and less at the mercy of your illness is one of the biggest and best benefits of becoming an exercise self-manager.

Developing an Active Lifestyle

Okay, so you want to be more physically active. One way is to set aside a special time for a formal exercise program involving walking, jogging, swimming, tennis, aerobic dance, an exercise videotape, and so on. But don't underestimate the value and importance of just being more physically active throughout the day as you carry out your usual activities. Both can be helpful.

The more formal programs are usually more visible and get more attention. But being more physical in everyday life can also pay off. Consider taking the stairs a floor or two instead of waiting impatiently for a slow elevator. Park and walk several blocks to work or to the store instead of circling the parking lot like a vulture looking for the perfect, up-close parking space. Mow the lawn. Work in the garden. These types of daily activities, often not viewed as "exercise," can add up to significant health benefits. Recent studies show that even small amounts of daily activity can raise fitness levels, improve strength, and boost mood . . . and the activities can be pleasurable, enjoyable ones! Dance, garden, play frisbee, golf . . . all these enjoyable activities can make a big difference. One patient commented that she *never* exercised. When asked why she went dancing several times a week she replied, "Oh, that's not exercise, that's fun." The average day is filled with excellent opportunities to be more physical.

Developing an Exercise Program

Although you can get lots of exercise from the activities of daily life, for many people, a more formal exercise program can be helpful. Such a program usually involves setting aside a period of time, at least several times a week, to deliberately focus on increasing fitness.

A complete, balanced exercise program should include the following three aspects of fitness:

- *Flexibility.* Flexibility refers to the ability of the joints to move through a full, normal range of motion. Limited flexibility can cause pain, increase risk of injury, and make muscles less efficient. Flexibility tends to decrease with age and certain diseases, but you can increase or maximize your flexibility by gentle stretching exercises.

- *Strength.* Muscles need to be exercised to maintain their strength. With inactivity, they tend to weaken and shrink (atrophy). The weaker the muscles get, the less we feel like using them and the more inactive we tend to become, creating a vicious circle. Much of the disability and lack of mobility in people with chronic illness is due to muscle weakness. This weakness can be reversed with a program of gradually increasing exercise.

- *Endurance.* Our ability to sustain activity depends on certain vital capacities. The heart and lungs must work efficiently to distribute oxygen-rich blood to the muscles. The muscles must be conditioned to extract and utilize the oxygen. Aerobic (meaning "with oxygen") exercise enhances cardiovascular (involving the heart and blood vessels) conditioning. This type of exercise uses the large muscles of your body in a rhythmical, continuous activity. The most effective activities involve your whole body: walking, swimming, dancing, mowing the lawn, and so on. Aerobic exercise improves cardiovascular fitness, lessens heart attack risk, and helps control weight. Aerobic exercise also promotes a sense of well-being . . . easing depression and anxiety, promoting restful sleep, and improving mood and energy levels.

A Good Fitness Program

A complete fitness program combines activities to improve each of the three aspects of fitness: flexibility, strength, and endurance. Exercise programs can be divided into three phases: (1) a warm-up, (2) an aerobic exercise or more vigorous conditioning period; and (3) a cool-down period. If you haven't exercised regularly in some time or have pain, stiffness, shortness of breath, or weakness that interferes with your daily activities, you should begin your fitness program with just the flexibility and strengthening warm-up, getting ready for more vigorous conditioning exercises at the next stage. If you have severe limitations, you may need to limit your fitness program to warm-up exercises only.

The Warm-Up

A warm-up routine consists of flexibility and strengthening exercises and a gradual increase in your activity level. It raises the temperature in your muscles and joints, nourishes joints, and safely prepares your heart and lungs to work harder during the exercise period. Maintaining flexibility and strength is vital for everyone, particularly people with chronic disease. A warm-up routine, therefore, should always be an important part of your exercise program.

For people with severe limitations, warm-up exercises may be all they do, and that's okay! You can have positive health benefits from a limited exercise program, too.

Always do flexibility and strengthening exercises before your exercise period. On some days, however, you may want to do only the gentle warm-up exercises and not the more vigorous exercise. Doing some flexibility exercises at least three times a week helps you keep the exercise habit and maintain optimal flexibility.

Choose a variety of flexibility and strengthening exercises. Start with 3 to 5 repetitions of your chosen exercises, exercising for a total of 1 to 10 minutes. Each week, add a few exercises and increase repetitions until you are doing flexibility and strengthening exercises for 5 to 15 minutes at a time. You can also get the benefits of 15 minutes of exercise, for example, by doing 1 minute

---

Helpful Tips for Doing Flexibility and Strengthening Exercises

- *Move slowly and gently.* Do not bounce or jerk. Those movements actually tighten and shorten muscles.

- To loosen tight muscles and limber up stiff joints, *stretch just until you feel tension*, hold for 5 to 10 seconds, and then relax.

- *Don't push your body until it hurts.* Stretching should feel good, not painful.

- *Start with no more than 5 repetitions of any exercise.* Take at least 2 weeks to increase to 10.

- *Arrange your exercises* so you don't have to get up and down off the floor a lot.

- Always do the *same number* of exercises for your left side as for your right.

- *Breathe naturally.* Do not hold your breath. Count out loud to make sure you are breathing easily.

- If you feel increased symptoms that last more than *2 hours* after exercising, next time do fewer repetitions, or eliminate an exercise that seems to be causing the symptoms. *Don't quit exercising.*

- *All exercises can be adapted for individual needs.* If you are limited by muscle weakness or joint tightness, go ahead and do the exercise as completely as you can. The benefit of doing an exercise comes from moving toward a certain position, not from being able to complete the movement perfectly the first time. In some cases you may find that after a while you can complete the movement. Other times you will continue to perform your own version.

each hour, or 2 minutes every other hour. Depending on your needs, you can choose a combination of exercises that include all parts of your body. Another approach is to work on particular body areas, changing exercises as needed. Before exercising a particular body area, be sure to flex and strengthen that area first. Ask a physical therapist for specific suggestions.

You might enjoy creating a routine of warm-up exercises that flow together. Arrange them so you don't have to get up and down off the floor often. Exercising to gentle, rhythmical music can also add to your enjoyment. When you can comfortably do 15 minutes of strengthening and flexibility exercises, you're ready to add 5 to 10 minutes of more vigorous aerobic conditioning, followed by a cool-down period.

Aerobic (Endurance) Exercise

There are many kinds of aerobic exercise. They all involve continuous rhythmic movement of the large muscles of the body at a sustained level of intensity. Walking, swimming, bicycling, and aquatic exercise are popular examples of aerobic activities especially suitable for people with chronic disease. But there are many more. Dancing, gardening, mowing the lawn, and even housework will qualify as long as you keep moving for at least 10 to 12 minutes at a time. Under "Exercising for Endurance," below, we describe how to gradually build up the time you can keep moving and how to monitor the intensity of the exercise.

The Cool-Down Period

A short 5- to 10-minute cool-down period after you have finished a vigorous activity is important to help your body gradually relax again. The cool-down allows your heart to slow gradually, lets your body lose some of the heat you generated during exercise, and gives your muscles a chance to relax and stretch out. Cooling down helps reduce the muscle soreness and stiffness that sometimes follows vigorous activity.

To cool down, continue your aerobic exercise in "slow motion" for 3 to 5 minutes. For example, after a brisk walk, cool down with a casual stroll. End a bicycle ride with slow, easy pedaling. It is also good to do some flexibility exercises because your muscles and joints are now warm. If you have been walking or bicycling, be sure to include an exercise to stretch the Achilles tendon (lower calf and ankle area of the leg). On days that you decide to do only light warm-up exercises, you may still include your cool-down routine.

Exercising for Endurance—
How Much Is Enough?

One of the biggest problems with endurance (aerobic) exercise is that it is easy to overdo, even for people who don't have HIV/AIDS. Inexperienced and misinformed exercisers think they have to work very hard for exercise to do any good. Exhaustion, sore muscles, painful joints, and shortness of breath are the results of jumping in too hard and too fast. As a result, some people may discontinue their exercise programs indefinitely, thinking that exercise is just not meant for them.

There is no magic formula for determining how much exercise you need. *The most important thing to remember is that some is better than none. Even a few minutes of exercise several times per week can be very beneficial.* If you start slowly and increase your efforts gradually, it is likely that you will maintain your exercise program as a lifelong habit. Generally it is better to begin your conditioning program by underdoing rather than overdoing.

Several studies suggest that the *upper* limit of benefit is about 200 minutes of moderate-intensity aerobic exercise per week. Doing more than that doesn't gain you much (and it increases your risk of injury). On the other hand, doing 100 minutes of exercise per week gets you about 90 percent of the gain, whereas 60 minutes of aerobic exercise per week yields about 75 percent of the gain. Sixty minutes is just 15 minutes of mild aerobic exercise 4 times a week!

Following are some general guidelines for the frequency, duration, and intensity of aerobic exercise.

- *Frequency.* Try to exercise three or four times a week. Taking every other day off gives your body a chance to rest and recover. We recommend that you rest at least one day per week.

- *Duration.* Start with just a few minutes, then gradually increase the duration of your aerobic activity to about 30 minutes a session. You can safely increase the time by alternating intervals of brisk exercise with intervals of rest or easy exercise. For example, after 3 to 5 minutes of brisk walking, do 1 to 2 minutes of easy strolling, then another 3 to 5 minutes of brisk walking. Eventually, you can build up to 30 minutes of activity. Then gradually eliminate rest intervals until you can maintain 20 to 30 minutes of brisk exercise. If 30 minutes seems too long, consider two sessions of 10–15 minutes each. Either way appears to improve fitness levels significantly.

- *Intensity.* Safe and effective endurance exercise should be done at no more than *moderate intensity.* High-intensity exercise increases the risk of injury and causes discomfort, so not many people stick with it. Exercise intensity is measured by how hard you work. For a trained runner, completing a mile in 12 minutes is probably low-intensity exercise. For a person who hasn't exercised in a long time, a brisk 10-minute walk may be of moderate to high intensity. For others with severe physical limitations, 1 minute may be of moderate intensity.

Remember, these are just rough guidelines on frequency, duration, and intensity, not a rigid prescription. Listen to your own body. Sometimes you need to tell yourself (and maybe others) that enough is enough. More exercise is not necessarily better, especially if it gives you pain or discomfort. As *The Walking Magazine* said, "Go for the smiles, not the miles."

You can determine your own individual intensity guidelines by several intensity-monitoring techniques: the talk test, perceived exertion, and heart rate. We discuss each of these below.

Talk Test

Talk to another person or yourself, sing, or recite poems out loud while you exercise. Moderate-intensity exercise allows you to speak comfortably. If you can't carry on a conversation or sing because you are breathing too hard or are short of breath, you're working too hard. Slow down. The talk test is an easy way to regulate exercise intensity.

If you have lung disease, the talk test might not work for you. If that is the case, try the perceived exertion test.

Perceived Exertion

Another way to monitor intensity is to rate how hard you're working on a scale of 0 to 10. Zero, at the low end of the scale, is lying down, doing no work at all. Ten is equivalent to working as hard as possible, very hard work that you couldn't do longer than a few seconds. Of course, you never want to exercise that hard. A good level for your aerobic exercise routine is between 3 and 6 on this scale. At this level, you'll usually feel sweaty, that you're breathing more deeply and faster than usual, and that your heart is beating faster than normal, but you should not be feeling pain.

Heart Rate

Monitoring your heart rate while exercising is one way to measure exercise intensity. The faster the heart beats, the harder you're working. (Your heart also beats fast when you are frightened or nervous, but here we're talking about how your heart responds to physical activity.) Endurance exercise at moderate intensity raises your heart rate into a range between 60 and 80 percent of your safe maximum heart rate. Safe maximum heart rate declines with age, so your safe exercise heart rate gets lower as you get older. You can follow the general guidelines of the Ideal Exercise Heart Rate chart below, or you can calculate your individual exercise heart rate. Either way, you need to know how to take your pulse.

Take your pulse by placing the tips of your middle three fingers at your wrist below the base of your thumb. Feel around in that spot until you feel the pulsations of blood pumping with each heartbeat. Count how many beats you feel in 15 seconds. Multiply this number by 4 to find out how fast your heart is beating in 1 minute. Start by taking your pulse whenever you think of it, and you'll soon learn the difference between your resting and exercise heart rates.

Ideal Exercise Heart Rate	
Age Range	*Exercise Pulse (15 sec)*
20–30	29–39
30–40	28–37
40–50	26–35
50–60	25–33
60–70	23–31
70–80	22–29
80+	16–24

How to calculate your own ideal exercise heart rate range:

1. Subtract your age from 220:

   Example: 220 − 40 = 180   You: 220 − _____ = _____

2. To find the *lower end* of your exercise heart rate range, multiply your answer in step 1 by 0.6.

   Example: 180 × 0.6 = 108   You: _____ × 0.6 = _____

3. To find the *upper end* of your exercise heart rate range, *which you should not exceed*, multiply your answer in step 1 by 0.8.

   Example: 180 × 0.8 = 144   You: _____ × 0.8 = _____

The exercise heart rate range in our example is from 108 to 144 beats per minute. What is yours?

Most people count their pulse for 15 seconds, not a whole minute. To find your 15-second pulse, divide both numbers by 4. The person in our example should be able to count between 24 and 32 beats in 15 seconds while exercising.

The most important reason for knowing your ideal exercise heart rate range is so that you can learn not to exercise too vigorously. After you've done your warm-up and 5 minutes of endurance exercise, take your pulse. If it's *higher than the upper rate, don't panic.* Slow down a bit. Don't work so hard.

At first, some people have trouble keeping their heart rate within the ideal exercise heart rate range. Don't worry about that. Keep exercising at the level with which you're most comfortable. As you get more experienced and stronger, you will gradually be able to do more vigorous exercise while keeping your heart rate within your "goal" range. But don't let the target heart rate monitoring become a burden. Recent studies have shown that even low-intensity exercise can provide significant health benefits. So use the ideal heart rate range as a rough guide, but don't worry if you can't reach the lower end of that range. The important thing is to keep exercising!

If you are taking medicine that regulates your heart rate, have trouble feeling your pulse, or think that keeping track of your heart rate is a bother, use one of the other methods to monitor your exercise intensity.

What Are Your Exercise Barriers?

Fitness makes sense. Yet, when faced with actually being more physically active, most people can come up with scores of excuses, concerns, and worries. These barriers can prevent us from even taking the first step. Following are some common barriers and possible solutions.

I don't have enough time.

Everyone has the same amount of time. We just choose to use it differently. It's a matter of priorities. Some find a lot of time for television, but nothing to spare for fitness. It doesn't really take a lot of time. Even 5 minutes a day is a good start, and much better than no physical activity. You may be able to combine activities, like watching television while pedaling a stationary bicycle, or arranging "walking meetings" to discuss business or family matters.

I'm too tired.

When you're out of shape, you feel listless and tend to tire easily. Then you don't exercise because you're tired, and this becomes a vicious cycle. You have to break out of the being-tired cycle. Regular physical activity increases your stamina and gives you more energy to do the things you like. As you get back into shape, you will recognize the difference between feeling listless or out of shape and feeling physically tired.

I'm too sick.

It may be true that you are too sick for a vigorous or strenuous exercise program, but you can usually find some ways to be more active. Remember, you can exercise 1 minute at a time, several times a day. The enhanced physical fitness you will gain can help you better cope with your illness and prevent further problems.

I get enough exercise.

This may be true, but for most people, their jobs and daily activities do not provide enough sustained exercise to keep them fully fit and energetic.

Exercise is boring.

You can make it more interesting and fun. Exercise with other people. Entertain yourself with a headset and musical tapes or listen to the radio. Vary your activities and your walking routes. Try to walk every street in your town by walking to a different place every day.

Exercise is painful.

The old saying "No pain, no gain" is simply wrong and out-of-date. Recent evidence shows significant health benefits come from gentle, low-intensity, enjoyable physical activity. You may sweat, or feel a bit short of breath, but if you feel more pain than before you started, something is probably wrong. More than likely you are either exercising improperly or you're overdoing it for your particular condition. Talk with your physician. You may simply need to be less vigorous or change the type of exercise that you're doing.

I'm too embarrassed.

For some, the thought of donning a skintight designer exercise outfit and trotting around in public is delightful, but for others it is downright distressing. Fortunately, as we'll describe, the options for physical activity range from exercise in the privacy of your own home to group social activities. You should be able to find something that suits you.

It's too cold, it's too hot, it's too dark . . .

If you are flexible, and vary your type of exercise, you can generally work around the changes in weather that make certain types of exercise more difficult. Consider indoor activities like a stationary bicycling or mall walking.

I'm afraid I won't be able to do it right or
be successful. I'm afraid I'll fail.

Many people don't start a new project because they are afraid they will fail or not be able to finish it successfully. If you feel this way about starting an exercise program, remember two things. First, whatever activities you are able to do—no matter how short or "easy"—will be much better for you than doing nothing. Be proud of what you *have* done, not guilty about what you *haven't* done. Second, new projects often seem overwhelming—until we get started and learn to enjoy each day's adventures and successes.

Perhaps you have come up with some other barriers. The human mind is incredibly creative. But you can turn that creativity to your advantage by using it to come up with even better ways to refute the excuses and develop positive attitudes about exercise and fitness. If you get stuck, ask others for suggestions, or try some of the self-talk suggestions in Chapter 5.

Preparing to Exercise

Figuring out how to make the commitment of time and energy to regular exercise is a challenge for everyone. If you have HIV/AIDS, you have even more challenges. You must take precautions and find a safe and comfortable program. Even with AIDS, most people can do some kind of aerobic exercise. If your illness is not fairly stable, if you have been inactive for more than 6 months, or if you have questions about starting an aerobic exercise program, it is best to check with your doctor or physical therapist first. Take this book with you when you discuss your exercise ideas, or prepare a list of your specific questions. If you have lung problems, you should generally not "exercise through" potentially serious symptoms, such as chest pain, shortness of breath, or excessive fatigue. You should notify your physician of any significant worsening of your usual symptoms or if new symptoms appear. Resumption of exercise should begin only after getting the physician's clearance to do so. Also, don't exercise when you are experiencing flu symptoms, an upset stomach, diarrhea, or other acute illnesses.

Learning how much to push yourself while exercising without doing "too much" is especially important. We hope that this chapter will help you gain knowledge to meet these challenges and enjoy the benefits of physical fitness. Start by learning your individual needs and limits. If possible, talk with your doctor and other health professionals. Get their ideas about special exercise needs and precautions. Learn to be aware of your body, and plan activities accordingly. Respect your body. If you feel acutely ill, don't exercise. If you can't comfortably complete your warm-up period of flexibility and strengthening exercises, then don't try to do more vigorous conditioning exercises. Your personal exercise program should be based on *your* current level of health and fitness, *your* goals and desires, *your* abilities and special needs, and *your* likes and dislikes. Deciding to improve your fitness and feeling the satisfaction of success have nothing to do with competition or comparing yourself with others.

Opportunities in Your Community

Most people who exercise regularly do so with at least one other person. Two or more people can keep each other motivated, and a whole class can build a feeling of camaraderie. On the other hand, exercising alone gives you the most freedom. You may feel that there are no classes that would work for you, or no buddy with whom to exercise. If so, start your own program; as you progress, you may find that these feelings change.

Many communities now offer a variety of exercise classes, including special programs for people with health problems, adaptive exercises, mall walking, fitness trails, and others. Check with the local Y, community centers, parks and recreation programs, adult education, and community colleges. There is a great deal of variation in the content of these programs, as well as in the professional experience of the exercise staff. By and large, the classes are inexpensive, and those in charge of planning are responsive to people's needs.

Health and fitness clubs usually offer aerobic studios, weight training, cardiovascular equipment, and sometimes a heated pool. For all these services they charge membership fees, which can be high. But some clubs have discounts for people with chronic illness. Ask about low-impact and beginners exercise classes, both in the aerobic studio and in the pool.* Gyms that emphasize weight lifting generally don't have the programs or personnel to help you with a flexible, overall fitness program.

In choosing an exercise class or a health and fitness club, look for the following qualities:

- Classes designed for *moderate- and low-intensity* exercise. You should be able to observe classes and participate in at least one class before signing up and paying.

- Instructors with *qualifications and experience*. Knowledgeable instructors are more likely to understand special needs and be willing and able to work with you.

- Membership policies that allow you to pay only for a session of classes, or let you "freeze" membership at times when you can't participate. Some fitness facilities offer *different rates* depending on how many services you use.

- Facilities that are *easy to get to, park near, and enter.* Dressing rooms and exercise sites should be accessible and safe, with professional staff on site.

- A pool that allows *"free swim"* times when the water isn't crowded. Also,

---

*You may be wondering whether it's safe for others if you use a public pool or exercise/fitness equipment. Are you putting other people at risk for catching HIV from you? Let's be clear here, because we don't want you avoiding exercise out of concern for others: *It is not dangerous for you to use public pools or exercise equipment or to play group sports.* No one has ever caught HIV from any kind of group sport or exercise. So just use normal sense. If you're bleeding, stop your exercise and clean up after yourself. Anyone should do the same, whether they have HIV or not.

find out the policy about children in the pool; small children playing and making noise may not be compatible with your program.

- Staff and other members whom you *feel comfortable* being around.

One last note: There are many excellent videotapes for home use. They vary in intensity from very gentle chair exercises to more strenuous aerobic exercise. Ask your doctor, physical therapist, or voluntary agency for suggestions, or review the tapes yourself.

Putting Your Program Together

The best way to enjoy and stick with your exercise program is to *suit yourself!* Choose what you want to do, a place where you feel comfortable, and an exercise time that fits your schedule. A young mother with school-age children will find it difficult to stick with an exercise program that requires her to leave home for a five o'clock class. A retired man who enjoys lunch with friends and an afternoon nap is wise to choose an early or midmorning exercise time.

Pick two or three activities you think you would enjoy and that wouldn't put undue stress on your body. Choose activities that can be easily worked into your daily routine. If an activity is new to you, try it out before going to the expense of buying equipment or joining a health club. By having more than one exercise, you can keep active while adapting to vacations, seasons, and changing problems with your illness. Variety also helps keep you from getting bored.

Having fun and enjoying yourself are benefits of exercise that often go unmentioned. Too often we think of exercise as serious business. However, most people who stick with a program do so because they enjoy it. *They think of their exercise as recreation rather than a chore*. Start off with success in mind. Allow yourself time to get used to new experiences, and you'll probably find that you look forward to exercise.

Some well-meaning health professionals can make it hard for a person with a chronic illness to stick to an exercise program. You may have been told simply to "exercise more" on your own. The how and when of that exercise plan, in fact, may have been left entirely up to you. No wonder so many people never start or give up so quickly! Not many of us would make a commitment to do something we don't fully understand. Experience, practice, and success help us establish a habit. Follow the self-management steps described in Chapter 2 to make beginning your program easier.

- *Choose exercises you want to do.* Combine any activities your doctor or another professional recommends with some of your favorites. You don't have to do the same thing every day. You can vary routines to make it more interesting. Write your exercise program down.
- *Choose the time and place to exercise.* Tell your family and friends your plan.
- *Make a contract with yourself.* Decide how long you'll stick with these particular exercises. Eight to 12 weeks is a reasonable time commitment for a new program.
- *Make an exercise diary* or calendar, leaving space to write down your exercises, how long you do them, your heart rate or perceived exertion score, and your feelings before and after exercise. We have included sample forms for an exercise diary at the end of this chapter. Put your diary where you can see it, and fill it out every day.
- *Do some self-tests.* Distance and time self-tests follow on page 103. Record the date and results. You may also use your exercise diary for this purpose.
- *Start your program.* Remember to begin gradually and proceed slowly, especially if you haven't exercised in a while.
- *Repeat the self-tests* at regular intervals, record the results, and check the changes.
- *Revise your program.* Look over your diary ideas. Decide what you liked, what worked, and what made exercising difficult. Modify your program and contract for another few weeks. You may decide to change some exercises, the place or time you exercise, or your exercise partners.
- *Reward yourself for a job well done.* Many people who start an exercise program find that the rewards come with improved fitness and endurance. Being able to enjoy family outings, a refreshing walk, or trips to a store, the library, a concert, or a museum are great rewards to look forward to.

Self-Tests for Endurance and Aerobic Fitness

For some people, just the feelings of increased endurance and well-being are enough to demonstrate progress. Others may find it helpful to demonstrate that their exercise program is making a measurable difference. You may wish to try one or both of these endurance and aerobic fitness tests before you start your exercise program. Not everyone will be able to do both the tests, so pick the one that works best for you. Record your results in your exercise diary. After 4 weeks of exercise, do the test again and check your improvement. Measure yourself again after 4 more weeks.

Distance Self-Test

- Find a place to walk or bicycle where you can measure distance. A running track works well. On a street you can measure distance with a car. A stationary bicycle with an odometer provides the equivalent measurement. If you plan on swimming, you can count pool lengths.

- After a warm-up, note your starting point and either bicycle, swim, or walk as briskly as you *comfortably* can for 5 minutes. Try to move at a steady pace for the full time. At the end of 5 minutes, mark your spot and immediately take your pulse and rate your perceived exertion from 0 to 10. Continue at a slow pace for 3 to 5 more minutes to cool down. Measure and record the distance, your heart rate, and your perceived exertion.

- Repeat the test after several weeks of exercise. There may be a change in as little as 4 weeks. However, it often takes 8 to 12 weeks to see improvement.

Goal: To cover more distance *or* to lower your heart rate *or* to lower your perceived exertion.

Time Self-Test

- Measure a given distance to walk, bike, or swim. Estimate how far you think you can go in 1 to 5 minutes. You can pick a number of blocks, actual distance, or lengths in a pool.

- Spend 3 to 5 minutes warming up. Start timing and start moving steadily, briskly, and comfortably. At the finish, record how long it took you to cover your course, your heart rate, and your perceived exertion.

- Repeat after several weeks of exercise. You may see changes in as soon as 4 weeks. However, it often takes 8 to 12 weeks for a noticeable improvement.

Goal: To complete the course in less time *or* at a lower heart rate *or* at a lower perceived exertion.

Maintaining Your Commitment to Exercise

If you haven't exercised recently, you'll undoubtedly experience some new feelings and discomfort in the early days. Most of these new feelings are normal and expected, but a few might mean you should change what you're doing. Look at the "Advice for Exercise Problems" on page 105 if you're concerned. But remember, it's normal to feel muscle tension and tenderness around joints, and to be a little more tired in the evenings. *Muscle or joint pain that lasts more than 2 hours after the exercise, or feeling tired into the next day, means that you probably did too much too fast. Don't stop;* just exercise less vigorously or for a shorter amount of time the next day.

When you do aerobic exercise, it's natural to feel your heart beat faster, your breathing speed up, and your body get warmer. However, irregular or very rapid heartbeats, excessive shortness of breath, or dizziness are not what you want. If this happens to you, stop exercising and discontinue your program until you check with your doctor.

Expect setbacks. During the first year of their exercise program, people average two to three interruptions in their exercise schedule, often because of minor injuries or illnesses unrelated to their exercise. You may find yourself sidelined or derailed temporarily. Don't be discouraged. Try a different activity or simply rest. When you are feeling better, resume your program, but begin at a lower, more gentle level. As a rule of thumb, it will take you the same amount of time to get back into shape as you were out. For instance, if you missed 3 weeks, it may take at least 3 weeks to get back to your previous level. Go slowly. Be kind to yourself. You're in this for the long haul.

Think of your head as the coach and your body as the team. For success, all parts of your team need attention. Be a good coach. *Encourage and praise yourself.* Design "plays" you feel your team can execute successfully. Choose places that are safe and hospitable. A good coach knows his or her team, sets good goals, and helps the team succeed. A good coach is loyal. A good coach does not belittle, nag, or make anyone feel guilty. Be a good coach to your team.

Besides a good coach, everyone needs an enthusiastic cheerleader or two. Of course, you can be your own cheerleader, but being both coach and cheerleader is a lot to do. Successful exercisers usually have at least one *family member* or *close friend who actively supports* their exercise habit. Your cheerleader can exercise with you, help you get chores done, praise your accomplishments, or just consider your exercise time when making plans. Sometimes cheerleaders pop up by themselves, but don't be bashful about asking for a hand.

With exercise experience you develop a sense of control over yourself and your chronic illness. You learn how to *alternate your activities to fit your day-to-day needs.* You know when to do less and when to do more. You know that a change in symptoms or a period of inactivity is usually only temporary and doesn't have to be devastating. You know you have the tools to get back on track again.

Give your exercise plan a chance to succeed. Set reasonable goals and enjoy your success. Stay motivated. When it comes to your personal fitness program, sticking with it and doing it your way makes you a definite winner.

Advice for Exercise Problems

Problem	Advice
Irregular or very rapid heartbeats	Stop exercising. Check your pulse. Are the beats regular or irregular? How fast is your heartbeat? Make a note of this information and discuss it with your doctor before exercising again.
Unusual, extreme shortness of breath, persisting 10 minutes after you exercise	Discuss with your doctor before exercising again.
Lightheadedness, dizziness, fainting, cold sweat, or confusion	Lie down with your feet up, or sit down and put your head between your legs. Talk to your doctor before you exercise again.
Excessive tiredness after exercise, especially if you're still tired 24 hours after you exercise	Don't exercise so vigorously next time. If the excessive tiredness persists, check with your doctor.

Resources

- Adult education
- Community colleges
- Health and fitness clubs
- Hospitals, health care organizations
- Parks and recreation programs
- YMCA, YWCA

Exercise Diary

Starting date _____   Ending date _____

Exercise Goals

1. _____
2. _____

Warm-Up *(Strengthening/flexibility)*	*Self-Test Score*		
	Time 1	*Time 2*	*Time 3*
1. _____			
2. _____			
3. _____			

Aerobic Exercise	*Time 1*	*Time 2*	*Time 3*
Activity _____			
Frequency _____			
Duration _____			
Exercise heart rate (EHR) _____			
Perceived exertion _____			

Cool-Down

1. _____
2. _____
3. _____

Exercise Diary (continued)					
Date	Exercise	Duration	EHR	Feelings Before	Feelings After

7

Eating Well

⎯⎯⎯

Eating well is important for all people, but it is especially essential for people with HIV/AIDS. Poor nutrition is common in people with HIV/AIDS. Sometimes it leads to a vicious cycle, with weight loss leading to decreased immune function, causing more infections, then poor food intake and digestion and more weight loss. But there is good news—although we don't have a cure for HIV/AIDS yet, we know a lot about how to prevent and improve the nutrition problems caused by HIV/AIDS. A good diet can help prevent the cycle of weight loss, help maintain and improve well-being, and contribute to quality of life. Having a good diet means eating a variety of foods so your body gets the appropriate amounts of all the nutrients it needs to function properly. It also means maximizing the pleasure and enjoyment of food, while coping with disease symptoms and maintaining a healthy weight.

In this chapter we discuss some important principles to consider when planning your diet. In Chapters 8 and 9 we offer simple ways to begin eating well and enjoy doing it. We will include tips for maintaining a healthy weight, changing eating patterns, and minimizing common eating problems of people with HIV/AIDS. Just as with any of the other self-management techniques discussed in this book, learning to eat well can help you feel more in control of your disease, and your life.

⎯⎯⎯⎯⎯⎯⎯

Portions of Chapters 7, 8, and 9 have been adapted from *Thinking About Losing Weight?*, Northern California Regional Health Education Center, Kaiser Permanente Medical Care Program, 1990; *The Weight Kit*, Stanford Center for Research in Disease Prevention, Health Promotion Resource Center, Stanford University, 1990; *Living Well With HIV and AIDS: A Guide to Healthy Eating*, American Dietetic Association, 1993; *HIV Disease Nutrition Guidelines*, Physicians Association for AIDS Care, 1993.

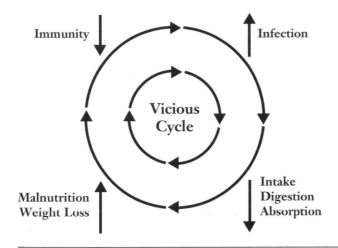

Figure 7.1   The Cycle of Poor Nutrition

What Is Healthy Eating?

Healthy eating means eating a *variety* of foods that you enjoy. No matter how "healthy" it may be, no single food is perfect. Each food has one or more important nutrients that your body needs. By choosing foods from all of the major food groups listed below, you ensure that you are getting all the nutrients you need for good health.

The Food Groups	
Protein	Meat, poultry, fish, eggs, dried beans and peas, nuts and seeds
Dairy	Milk, yogurt, cheese
Starches	Bread, cereal, rice, pasta
Fruits	Bananas, apples, grapes, oranges, grapefruit
Vegetables	Cabbage, broccoli, green peppers, mushrooms, zucchini, spinach, yams
Fats and sweets	Oil, butter, margarine, salad dressing, avocado, mayonnaise, candy

Are calories important?

Calories are the energy in food. They provide your body with fuel so it can keep running. If you eat the amounts of food you should every day, and eat different kinds of foods, you may not have to worry too much about calories. But sometimes your calorie needs may increase, such as during fever and infections.

If you are worried about getting enough calories, follow these easy guidelines to increase your caloric intake:

- Eat foods that you like.
- Try to eat frequent small meals (at least four or more times per day).
- Eat a variety of foods from each of the food groups.

What about other nutrients—are they important for health?

Yes! Nutrients are the parts of foods that your body uses to keep itself strong. Lots of nutrients are important for health, including fats, carbohydrates, water, protein, minerals, and vitamins.

How is water important for health?

Although many people don't think of it, water is a very important nutrient. Your body uses a lot of water each day, and you need to replace it. All foods contain water. Any drink (juice, regular soda pop, milk) and foods like soups, ice pops, and gelatin can help to replace water. But remember to choose drinks without caffeine or alcohol because these substances can actually *increase* water loss by stimulating urination.

What about protein?

Your muscles, organs, and many of the substances that make up your body's immune system are all made of proteins. When you don't get enough calories and protein in your food, your body uses its own protein (muscles) to make up for the lack of fuel. As a consequence, you may not have the energy and protein you need to stay healthy and keep your immune system working. The right amounts of calories and protein in combination give you energy to fight infections and form the strongest defense against losing muscle.

What should I eat to get enough protein?

Protein can come from animal products, like meat, fish, poultry, eggs, and dairy products. Or, you can get protein from dried beans and peas, nuts, vegetables, and grains. Peanuts, almonds, or sunflower seeds; peanut or other nut butters; cooked kidney beans, pinto beans, lentils, or split peas; and soy milk and tofu (soy bean curd) are good substitutes if you don't want to eat animal products. Some vegetables and grain products, such as wheat bread, pasta, barley, and rice, contain smaller amounts of protein.

Commercial products or supplements in powdered or liquid form also provide protein, carbohydrate, fat, vitamins, and minerals. Some have higher amounts of protein and calories than others, and some contain different forms of fat. These products can be used to boost the protein and calories in your diet or even replace meals when you're not feeling up to preparing food for yourself or eating out. Because of the variety of supplements available and because your individual needs will vary, it is best to talk to your dietitian or doctor to choose a product that is best for you.

How often should I eat?

Try to eat at least four times a day. People who eat four or more times per day usually have an easier time keeping their weight stable. Instead of three large meals, you can have one big meal and several smaller snacks or even six small meals. You may find that eating three meals and several small snacks each day works best. Each time you eat, try to include a variety of foods. Chapters 8 and 9 will help you learn how to plan a healthful diet that includes the five food groups.

Are there special things I should be eating to boost my immune system?

Research on nutrition and the immune system has shown that certain vitamins and minerals are important for good immune function. However, no one ingredient has been shown to be the "key ingredient," and no one diet is the "miracle diet." Anyone who says they *do* have a magic ingredient is probably trying to sell you something.

Following a healthy diet for HIV/AIDS is not complicated. Eat a variety of foods from each of the major food groups, and you will help *all* of the different systems of your body work well, including the immune system.

Am I getting enough vitamins and minerals?

Vitamin and mineral supplements can't take the place of a good balanced diet. If you're getting enough calories in a diet with a variety of foods from the groups listed above, you're probably getting enough minerals and vitamins.

Some nutrition and medical experts do suggest that people with HIV infection take a daily multivitamin and mineral supplement. These supplements come in a single tablet and contain vitamins and minerals in the amounts that you need on a daily basis. But again, they are not a substitute for foods. A vitamin and mineral pill and a cup of coffee, for example, is not a good breakfast. And remember, two pills are not necessarily better than one and may even be too much for you.

Which vitamin and mineral supplements should I take?

Choose a vitamin and mineral supplement that contains 100 percent to 200 percent of the U.S. RDA (Recommended Dietary Allowance) for vitamins and minerals. It is not a good idea to take supplements that contain large doses of vitamins or minerals unless you discuss them with your doctor. Overdoses of certain vitamins and minerals can cause serious side effects, such as nausea, diarrhea, and loss of appetite. Such overdoses can even damage your liver and kidneys.*

To summarize, the basic principles to eating well are simple. Chapters 8 and 9 will describe some ways to incorporate these principles into your diet.

Basic Principles of Eating Well

- Eat a *variety of foods* from each of the food groups every day.
- Eat enough *fresh fruits and vegetables* for vitamins and minerals.
- Eat *small, frequent meals* or snacks (at least four times per day).
- Include a good amount of *fluids* in your diet each day.
- If your weight is below normal, *increase your calories* by eating more starches, proteins, and fats.
- Take a *multivitamin/mineral supplement* each day.
- *Avoid chemical stimulants,* such as:
    caffeine (coffee, some dark teas, regular sodas)
    alcoholic drinks (beer, wine, whiskey, and others)
    recreational drugs (cigarettes, cigars, cocaine, marijuana, "speed," and others)

---

*Avoid taking high doses ("megadoses") of vitamins and minerals. Megadoses of many vitamins and minerals can cause toxic reactions. Megadosing is a type of drug therapy, and as such, needs medical supervision.

Suggested Reading

Physicians Association for AIDS Care (PAAC), *HIV Disease Nutrition Guidelines: Practical Steps for a Healthier Life.* Stadtlanders Pharmacy, 1-800-238-7828 to obtain copies for distribution. (A 21-page booklet containing recommendations from nutritionists experienced in HIV care. Topics include: advice on balancing food intake, exercise, and stress management, guidelines on managing side effects, and resource information for obtaining further advice, counseling, and support service.)

Resources

Nutrition

- Dietitian or nutritionist at your health care center
- Community food distribution programs (Meals on Wheels, Project Open Hand)

8

Making a Plan
for Healthy Eating

We all know that eating well is important. But it's hard to change eating habits! After all, eating is something each of us does every day throughout life. We all have habits for what we like to eat and for how, when, and where we like to eat. So even if a person knows she should change her eating, it's hard to know how to actually do it. Making plans is the essence of being a self-manager, so it's time to make a plan for healthy eating. This chapter takes you through the steps. Here's what you need to do:

- *Get motivated.* Sure, a better diet is a good idea in general, but how will it help me, specifically?
- *Make sure you're ready.* Change your diet when you have a good chance of succeeding.
- *Look at what you eat and what you want to change.* Keep track of what you're doing and make one change at a time.
- *Figure out the obstacles.* What are the things that are making it tough to eat better?

This is a framework for you to work with and change. *You* are the self-manager!

Why Change My Diet?

The reasons for changing eating habits are different for each individual. The most obvious reason may be your physical health, but you may also have psychological or emotional reasons for wanting to change. Examine for yourself why you want to change. You may want to change your eating habits in order to:

- lessen your disease symptoms, such as pain, fatigue, and shortness of breath
- have more energy to do the things you want to do
- feel better about yourself
- strengthen your resistance to infection
- change the way others perceive you
- feel more in control of your disease and your life

If you have other reasons, jot them down here:

_____

_____

_____

_____

Am I Ready to Change for Good?

If you have decided that you want to change, next consider if you are ready to make these changes for good. Remember, success is important. If you are not ready, you may be setting yourself up for failure and those nasty weight "ups and downs." This is not only discouraging but unhealthy. Therefore, try to plan ahead. Is there someone or something that will make it easier for you to change? Or, are there problems or obstacles that will keep you from becoming more active or changing the way you eat? Will worries or concerns about friends, work, or other commitments affect your ability to carry out your plans successfully? Looking ahead at these factors can help you find ways to build support for desired changes, as well as minimize possible problems you may encounter along the way. Use the Diet Change Readiness chart on the next page to help you identify some of these factors.

After you have examined the factors involved in your making a diet change, you may find that now is not the right time to start anything. If it is not, set a date in the future for a time when you will reevaluate these changes. In the meantime, accept that this is the right decision for you at this time, and focus your attention on other goals.

If you decide that now *is* the right time, start by changing those things that feel most *comfortable to you*. You don't have to do it all right away. Remember, slow and steady wins the race.

Diet Change Readiness	
Things That Will Help Me to Make the Desired Changes	*Things That Will Make It Difficult for Me to Change*
Example: I have the support of family and friends.	*Example:* I like to go out with my friends, and the places we go only serve junk food and alcohol.

What Will I Have to Change?

We've already looked at some of the components of a healthy diet in Chapter 6. Let's get more specific. Remember, the recipe for healthy eating is simple: a variety of foods that contain calories, protein, and other nutrients. Combine with plenty of fluids, and serve in a pleasant atmosphere. Making changes in your eating patterns does not mean following a rigid diet; it starts by making *small, gradual changes* in what you eat. This may mean changing the emphasis or quantity of certain foods you eat.

To help get started, *keep track of what you are currently doing.* Start with yesterday. List each food you ate and the amount under the food group categories in a food diary like the one at the end of this chapter. For mixed dishes like pizza or spaghetti, estimate how much of each food group your serving had in it. By using the portion sizes described below, check off the minimum number of servings that you ate from each food group to see how your diet measures up.

Now you can begin to plan changes. Use the food groups as a guide to planning a healthful diet. To maintain the balance of nutrients you need for good health, remember you will need a minimum number of servings from each food group.

Protein: meat, poultry, fish, eggs, dried beans and peas, nuts and seeds

You will need at least 3 servings each day. A serving is:

- 2 to 3 ounces of cooked meat, fish, or poultry
- 2 cooked eggs
- 4 tablespoons of peanut butter (or other nut butter)
- 1 cup of cooked dried beans or peas
- 1/2 cup of nuts or seeds
- 5 to 6 ounces of tofu

Dairy: milk, yogurt, and cheese

You will need at least 3 servings each day. A serving is:

- 1 cup milk
- 1 cup yogurt
- 1 cup of ice cream or frozen yogurt
- 1 cup of cooked dried beans or peas
- 1/2 cup of cottage cheese
- 1 to 2 ounces of cheese

Starches: bread, cereal, rice, and pasta

You will need 8 to 11 servings each day. A serving is:

- 1 slice of bread
- 1/2 of an English muffin, bagel, or bun
- 1 cup of flake-type cereal
- 1/2 cup of cooked cereal
- 1/2 cup of cooked pasta or rice
- 2 flour or corn tortillas
- 6 saltine-type crackers
- 3 squares graham crackers

Fruits

You will need at least 3 servings each day. A serving is:

- 1 medium-sized apple, banana, orange, or other whole fruit (washed well or peeled)
- 1/2 cup of chopped, cooked, or canned fruit
- 3/4 cup of fruit juice
- 1/4 cup of dried fruit

Vegetables

You will need at least 4 servings each day. A serving is:

- 1 cup of raw leafy vegetables (washed thoroughly)
- 1/2 cup of other vegetables, cooked or chopped raw (washed thoroughly)
- 3/4 cup of vegetable juice

Fats and sweets

Foods that are high in fat—such as margarine, salad dressings, sour cream, and mayonnaise—can be added to foods for flavor and to boost the amount of calories you eat. Sweet foods like sugar, jelly, jam, honey, and syrup also can be added for extra calories.

How Do I Get Started?

Sometimes getting started is the hardest part. *Make one change at a time.* You may decide to change *how* you eat before you change *what* you eat. If you skip meals now, it might be a good idea to start by eating more regularly. After you get into the habit of eating four or more times a day, you might make other changes, such as adding more cereal and bread to your diet or eating more fruits and vegetables.

The key is planning. Decide which foods you *want* to eat. Then begin planning a daily menu that uses those foods. Fill in your menu with foods from food groups you missed to make your diet complete. The sample menu below can serve as a good starting point.

Sample Menu—Be Creative!	
Morning	*Midmorning Snack*
Apricot nectar Scrambled eggs with cheese Toast with margarine Honey or jelly Hot cocoa with added nonfat dry milk	Hot or cold cereal with raisins Half and half, whole milk, or milk substitute
Midday	*Midafternoon Snack*
Cream of vegetable soup Turkey sandwich with mayonnaise, lettuce, and tomato Cookies Whole milk	Fruit yogurt Graham crackers
Evening	*Evening Snack*
Salad with dressing Meat lasagna Zucchini Dinner roll Fruit juice Apple pie	Peanut butter and crackers Canned peaches

Common Obstacles to Changing Eating Habits

Whether your goal is weight management or just eating for good nutrition, changing old eating habits is no easy task. No matter how much you want to change, there's always something that gets in the way. In the next section we've listed some of the most common barriers encountered by people and some strategies for dealing with them. This can be your starting point as you find out what your own barriers are and how you're going to overcome them.

What if I'm not getting enough of one of the food groups?

Then it's time to make a better eating plan. Build an eating plan that's *right for you.* Set up a plan that meets your needs whether you eat at home, at work, at restaurants, or have food brought to your house. If you're not getting enough food from one of the groups, don't panic—there are many different ways to eat healthily.

I eat out a lot. Sometimes I can't get any fruit or vegetables.

Most restaurants offer a wide variety of foods. Even fast-food restaurants have salads, milk, and other nutritious choices. If you can't eat from all of the food groups, fill in the missing food groups with snacks from home—for example, fresh fruit, vegetable juices, and crackers with peanut butter. Keep your refrigerator and cupboard stocked with snacks like these.

I know some foods are good for me, but I just don't like them.

Each of the food groups has many different nutrients, so you can find substitutes for the foods you don't like or don't want to eat. If you don't like a certain food, try choosing another food in the same group. If you don't like an entire food group, you may need to consult with a dietitian to find foods from other groups that can give you similar nutrients.

I don't like vegetables.

Try raw vegetables with tasty dips or sauces to add flavor. Grated or frozen vegetables can be used in soups, stews, or meat loaf. Choose vegetable casseroles, like vegetable lasagna. If vegetables still don't appeal to you, increase the fruits and breads you eat.

I don't like to drink milk.

Instead of drinking milk, add it (or dry milk powder) to foods like soups, meat loaf, or casseroles. You can also choose pudding, yogurt, cottage cheese, or ice cream in place of milk. Try yogurt in a salad dressing or in a vegetable or fruit dip. Try melting cheese on vegetables, potatoes, beans, tortillas, in a grilled cheese sandwich, on pizza, or in a dip. To get some of the same nutrients that are in milk without eating cheese or yogurt, try broccoli, greens (such as kale or collard or beet greens), tofu, beans, canned salmon, and corn tortillas. If milk or milk products make you feel bloated and cause diarrhea or gas, see the section on dairy products and lactose intolerance in Chapter 9.

I'm a vegetarian. I don't want to eat any animal foods.

You can be a vegetarian and still have an excellent diet. To make sure you get the protein and other nutrients usually supplied by food from animals, include fortified soybean milk, tofu, beans, and other plant protein sources along with a variety of breads, grains, pasta, beans, fruits, and vegetables. If meat, fish, and poultry are the only animal foods you don't eat, include a variety of dairy products and eggs, in addition to breads, grains, pastas, beans, and tofu.

I'd rather eat sweets and snack foods like chips,
candy, and cookies.

You can include these foods in your meals and snacks; in fact, they are important sources of calories. But try to eat foods from each of the food groups first. If you're still hungry, or if you have a taste for more, then add your favorite sweets and snack foods. Try not to let chips, candy, and cookies take the place of other foods that supply important nutrients.

It takes too long to prepare meals. By the time I'm done,
I'm too tired to eat!

You need to eat to maintain your energy level. If meal preparation is a problem for you, it's time to develop a plan. Here are some energy-saving tips:

- Plan your meals for the week.
- Then go to the grocery store and buy everything you will need.
- Break your food preparation into steps, resting in between.
- Cook enough for two, three, or even more servings, especially if it's something you really like.
- Freeze the extra portions in single-serving sizes. On the days when you are really tired, thaw and reheat one of these precooked frozen meals.
- Ask for help, especially for big meals or at social gatherings.

I've never really been a cook, and I can't start now.

Keep it simple. Keep your freezer stocked with prepared meals: pizzas, vegetables, and other convenience foods. Try easy-to-prepare meals like a grilled cheese sandwich and canned soup, eggs and toast, cereal and milk, or macaroni and cheese. Go to the public library and look through some cookbooks to get ideas for quick meals. When you do cook, make larger amounts and freeze portions to heat up later.

Changing your eating habits is not easy, and the suggestions given here are only a start. But the key to changing how you eat is in the overall approach: make sure you're motivated, figure out what you're doing now, figure out some practical "do-able" changes you can make, and solve any problems that come up. These steps really can be applied to all kinds of changes you might want to make, and good self-managers use them all the time.

Suggested Reading

Living Well With HIV and AIDS: A Guide to Healthy Eating. American Dietetic Association, 1993. (An excellent summary.)

Food Diary		
Food Group	*Foods Eaten*	*Minimum No. of Servings*
Protein meat, poultry, fish, eggs, dried beans and peas, nuts and seeds		*3 or more*
Dairy milk yogurt cheese		*3 or more*
Starches bread cereal rice pasta		*8 or more*
Fruits bananas, apples, grapes, oranges, grapefruit		*3 or more*
Vegetables cabbage, broccoli, green peppers, mushrooms, zucchini, spinach, yams		*4 or more*
Fats and Sweets oil, butter, margarine, salad dressing, avocado, mayonnaise, candy		

9

Eating Problems and Food Safety

Like everyone, people with HIV/AIDS want to eat a generally healthy diet that tastes good and makes them feel good. But people with HIV/AIDS are faced with two specific problems that aren't as common in other people. The first problem is maintaining a healthy body weight. Not everyone loses weight, but certainly many people do. Weight loss can happen for all kinds of reasons, but the solution is always to find a way to put more calories into the body than the body burns up.

People with HIV/AIDS always need to avoid infections, so the second problem is making sure there's no contamination when buying, storing, and preparing food. We'll look at both these problems in this chapter.

Managing Eating Problems

The symptoms that you experience from an infection, from depression, or as a side effect to treatment may determine how you feel about eating. But eating a variety of foods combined with keeping your weight at a proper level will help strengthen your body and its ability to fight infection. *Weight loss is a warning signal that means you're not providing your body with enough calories.* Never ignore weight loss, even if it happens gradually. Talk with your doctor to determine possible causes of weight loss. But what kinds of problems make eating difficult?

I don't feel like eating anything.

Loss of appetite is a common problem that can be caused by medication, fatigue, concern about your illness, or an infection. On days when you feel like eating, be sure to eat plenty to make up for days when your appetite is bad. When you are having trouble with poor appetite, the following suggestions can help you get the calories you need:

- Eat smaller amounts more frequently if you don't feel like having a large meal.
- Eat in a relaxed setting, with a friend, or while listening to your favorite music.
- Eat your favorite foods as often as you like.
- Add more flavor to your foods with spices and herbs, lemon wedges, mustard, barbecue sauce, catsup, or hot sauce.
- Order take-out food delivered to your home, or check in your area for home food delivery services, such as Project Open Hand or Meals on Wheels.
- Keep a snack supply of high-calorie, high-protein foods, such as crackers, cheese, peanut butter, and ice cream. Eat them whenever you feel like it.
- Liquid foods or foods that do not take a lot of energy to chew or cook are perfect for times like this. When you don't feel like eating much, make a milkshake or have a supplement drink. (Your doctor, nurse, or dietitian can recommend one.)
- Try not to fill up on liquids before you eat. Drink small amounts when you eat and sip fluids between your eating times.
- Keep easy-to-prepare foods on hand for quick fixing, such as canned food, frozen meals, or frozen leftovers.

It's important to consume enough calories and nutrients to avoid weight loss. If you find that you can't keep your appetite up, consult your doctor. He or she can refer you to a dietitian, who can help you plan meals that maximize the value of what you eat. The doctor can also prescribe appetite stimulants if needed. So be sure to mention it to your doctor if your appetite is decreasing and you seem to be losing weight.

I get full too fast.

Eat often during the day. Three meals a day may not be enough for you, especially if you can't eat a full meal at one sitting. Eating five to six times per day seems to work best for most people with HIV/AIDS, particularly those who do not feel well. Make what you eat count: choose foods with lots of calories and protein to help meet your need for these important nutrients.

Food doesn't taste as good as before.

Some medications can cause changes in taste sensations, or an overall decrease. Being on oxygen can also cause taste problems. Try one or more of the following suggestions to enhance the flavor of food:

- Experiment with herbs, spices, and other seasonings. Start with just about 1/4 teaspoon in a dish that serves four.
- Modify recipes to include a wide variety of ingredients to make the food look and taste more appealing.
- Chew your food well. This will allow the food to remain in your mouth longer and provide more stimulation to your taste buds.

If you are having trouble eating enough for any reason, try to pack more calories and protein into your food with some of the ideas in the following box.

Getting More Calories and Protein

Add	*To*
Butter, margarine, sour cream	Vegetables, cooked cereal, potatoes, noodles, or rice
Dried fruits or nuts, honey, jam, sugar, cream, half and half	Hot or cold cereal
Bacon, avocado, olives, mayonnaise	Sandwiches, salads, or casseroles
Cream or sour cream	Soups, fruit, or puddings
Cream cheese	Fruit or crackers
Peanut butter	Sauces, shakes, toast, crackers, waffles, or celery
Extra chopped meat, shredded cheese, hard-cooked eggs, egg substitutes	Soups, sauces, vegetables, salads, and casseroles
Dry milk powder	Regular milk, scrambled eggs, soups, gravies, or desserts

When I eat, I feel like I'm going to throw up.

An infection or a medication side effect can cause nausea, making foods just not seem appealing.

The following suggestions may lessen feelings of nausea when you eat:

- Salty foods or dry foods such as bread or crackers may help to calm your stomach.

- Cold foods such as ice cream, frozen yogurt, sherbet, gelatin, pudding or custard, cottage cheese and fruit, ice pops, juice, cold cereal, or a sandwich may be easier to eat.

- Eating small, frequent meals is a good idea. Often, nausea is worse when there is nothing in your stomach.

- Rest between your meals, but do not lie completely flat. Elevate your upper body or sit up for at least 2 hours after eating.

- If the smell of food bothers you, ask someone to cook for you or make sure that the cooking area is well ventilated so that food smells don't linger.

- Spicy foods, high-fat foods, and caffeine may be hard to tolerate and also can be irritating to your stomach or intestines.

- If your medication seems to cause nausea, check with your doctor or pharmacist to time your doses so that you can take them when you are eating or right after you eat.

Diarrhea is a problem for me.

Diarrhea can be caused by many things, including medications, stress, infections, or severe weight loss. Whatever the cause, diarrhea means that your body is not getting the important nutrients from the foods you are eating. It is also critical that you pay attention to your fluid intake to prevent dehydration.

The following tips will help you deal with and lessen your diarrhea:

- Drink plenty of liquids, such as juices, clear carbonated beverages, broth, fruit drinks, sports beverages, or water. It is best to avoid drinks containing caffeine or alcohol; they are stimulating to the intestines, and alcohol can cause further dehydration. Try frozen liquids such as ice pops or sherbet. Gelatin counts as a liquid and may be a food that is easy to eat.

- Potassium is a vital mineral that is lost when you have diarrhea, and depletion can lead to muscle cramping and fatigue. Replace lost potassium with bananas, sports drinks, fruit juices (especially orange juice and nectars), mashed potatoes, or canned fruits without seeds or skins.

- You may not feel like eating much, but skipping meals is not a good idea. Foods you may be able to tolerate are plain white rice, noodles, mashed potatoes, crackers, white toast, eggs, hot cereal, applesauce or other canned fruits without seeds or skins, bananas, gelatin, ice cream, sherbet, or broth-type soups.

- Avoid greasy or fatty foods with excessive amounts of butter, margarine, or oils, and foods that are fried. For more tips, see the section on fat intolerance below.

- Foods that are high in fiber or that have skins or seeds can be irritating and are also hard to digest. Avoid raw fruits and vegetables and whole-grain breads or cereals. Cooked vegetables, canned fruits without skins and seeds, and white bread are better choices when diarrhea is a problem.

- You can eat low-fat milk and lean meats if you can tolerate them. Dairy aids containing lactase can help you digest and absorb the milk sugar that causes some people problems such as bloating and diarrhea (see the section on lactose intolerance below). Stick to plain boiled, baked, or broiled meats, and stay away from spicy foods or sauces.

- Cramps often accompany diarrhea and can be a sign of gas or air in your intestines. Drinking carbonated beverages can worsen this problem and should be avoided. Foods that cause gas, such as beans, cabbage, broccoli, cauliflower, or brussels sprouts, should also be avoided if they seem to cause these problems.

Note: If your diarrhea increases in frequency or lasts for more than a week, consult your doctor. Unchecked diarrhea can cause further problems, and medications to help you get it under control are available. Dehydration and potassium loss are the serious problems that must be prevented or corrected. (See Chapter 3 for more information about evaluating diarrhea.)

I have trouble digesting fat (fat intolerance).

Fats are an excellent source of calories. They can also be hard to digest at times. Fat intolerance—difficulty digesting and absorbing fats—can be a problem for people with HIV infection and AIDS. If you feel discomfort after eating a meal or a food that was high in fat, you may need to reduce the amount of fat you eat. You usually do not have to cut it completely from your

Foods High in Fat

- Fried foods
- Chips
- Tuna in oil
- French fries
- Salad dressing
- Chocolate
- Rich desserts
- Too much butter, oil, or margarine
- Mayonnaise
- Pepperoni
- Cheeses
- Cream sauces
- Hot dogs
- Ice cream
- Sausages
- Cream or half and half
- Whole milk
- Luncheon meats
- Bacon
- Gravies
- Peanut butter
- Doughnuts

diet. In fact, this is not usually recommended unless you are experiencing prolonged and severe diarrhea. If fat intolerance becomes a problem, it is best to avoid fat-rich foods, like the ones listed in the table above.

If your problem with fat is very severe, products that contain no fat but have extra calories and protein are available. And some products have a special, easily digestible form of fat. These products may be helpful to keep your intake and weight at appropriate levels.

I don't feel well when I eat dairy products (lactose intolerance).

If you notice that milk, cheese, and ice cream cause cramping, gas, bloating, or diarrhea, your body may be having trouble digesting lactose, a type of sugar found in milk and milk products. You may find that suddenly you cannot tolerate dairy products of any kind, but with time your reactions may subside and you can add these dairy foods—which are good protein sources—back into your diet.

If you experience problems with milk or other dairy products, the following suggestions should help you avoid the more troublesome dairy products and find ones you may be able to tolerate:

- Beware of foods containing milk, such as pudding, custard, ice cream, cream soups, cream pies, gravies, or sauces, as they may also cause problems.

- Products are available that contain an enzyme called *lactase*, which will help you digest lactose. Lactase pills and drops should be taken before you eat something that contains large amounts of lactose. Some milk and dairy food items already have these products in them and are found in the regular dairy section of your supermarket.

- Some dairy products contain less lactose and therefore may be easier to tolerate. Buttermilk, cottage cheese, sour cream, aged cheeses, sherbet, and yogurt are examples. In place of milk, try nondairy products like enriched soy milk, nondairy cream, or other milk substitutes.
- Kosher foods labeled *pareve* or *parve* are acceptable because they are milk-free.

Mouth sores, dry mouth, and swallowing problems make it hard to eat anything.

Infections in your mouth and throat can cause painful sores, making it difficult to eat or swallow. Some medications can also make your mouth feel dry. Taking care of your teeth and gums is important and often can help you manage these symptoms.

The following suggestions will help you find foods you can eat:

- Soft foods that are smooth in consistency and easy to swallow are usually the easiest to eat. You can make swallowing easier by putting food through a blender, eating casseroles and stews, adding gravies or sauces to finely cut meat, or choosing dishes that don't have chunks of food in them. Adding liquids to foods or dunking foods in liquids can make them less irritating to your mouth and throat.
- Avoid spicy foods, extremely hot foods, or foods with a high acid content, such as orange juice or tomatoes; they can make mouth sores more painful. Cold foods such as ice pops, ice cream, sherbet, frozen yogurt, or thick milkshakes can numb your mouth and can be easy to swallow as well.
- If you find that you gag easily, avoid sticky foods, such as peanut butter, and slippery foods, such as gelatin.
- Sometimes food that is neither too hot nor too cold is easier to handle. Try puddings, custard, eggs, canned fruits, cottage cheese, yogurt, bananas, and creamed cereals. Or try dipping toast, cookies, or crackers in milk or another beverage.
- Avoid foods that require a lot of chewing or are tough and fibrous.
- Rinse your mouth frequently and drink lots of fluid to help with dryness. If dryness continues to be a problem even when you moisten your foods, your doctor or dentist may prescribe artificial saliva for you.

Should a fever change my eating?

Your needs for both fluid and calories are higher when you have a fever. Fevers or night sweats may not affect how you feel about eating, but if you are experiencing either of these symptoms, remember to drink more fluids (more than 8 cups per day) and eat frequently, up to six or more times daily if you can. This is also an important time to watch your weight closely, as it can signal whether you're getting enough nutrients from your food.

Food Safety

Food poisoning, which can occur when you eat foods containing large amounts of harmful bacteria, is of special concern to people with HIV/AIDS. It can cause nausea, vomiting, and diarrhea, all of which can make you miserable, and it can also interfere with eating and lead to weight loss. It is important to pay careful attention to food safety when shopping, preparing, serving, and storing foods, as well as when eating away from home. The American Dietetic Association has recommended the following precautions to ensure food safety:

Shopping

- Check the dates on food containers. Don't buy or use packaged food past the recommended date on the label.
- Shop for cold and frozen foods last and ask that these foods be packed in the same bag.
- Carry a cooler in the car to store cold and frozen foods if the trip home is longer than 30 minutes.
- Check your own refrigerator occasionally for foods that are past their expiration dates.

Storage

- Proper storage of foods is a key step to ensuring food safety. Be sure to refrigerate or freeze foods that need cold storage as soon as possible after buying them. Cold foods should be stored in a refrigerator that is 40°F or lower, and frozen foods in a freezer that is 0°F or lower. Use a refrigerator thermometer to make sure the temperatures are in the proper range.

- Label your stored foods with the date of purchase and follow suggested storage times for each type of food. Remember that foods containing harmful bacteria will not always look or smell spoiled. When in doubt, throw it out.
- Always thaw frozen foods in the refrigerator or microwave oven and place leftover prepared foods containing meat, eggs, or milk products in the refrigerator or freezer immediately.
- Use refrigerated foods within the time limits shown to keep them from spoiling or becoming dangerous to eat.

Preparation

- Always begin by washing your hands with soapy water. Also, be sure to wash your hands after handling any raw foods and before handling cooked foods.
- Care of cooking and eating utensils is also important. Cutting boards and chipped china or crockery can collect bacteria that cause infection and always should be cleaned in a dishwasher or washed in hot (at least 140°F), soapy water and rinsed well. After working with raw meats, fish, and poultry, it's a good idea to sanitize your cutting board by soaking it for 10 minutes in a mixture of 1 teaspoon of bleach per gallon of warm water. Clean counter tops with this same sanitizing solution as an additional safety step.

Meat, poultry, and fish

- Never consume raw meat, poultry, or fish of any kind. Even steak tartare, carpaccio, raw oysters, raw shrimp, sashimi, or sushi topped with raw fish can cause serious infections.
- Cook all meats to 165°F or higher. Cook poultry to 180°F. Use a meat thermometer to be sure that a safe temperature is reached.
- Never thaw frozen meats or foods containing dairy products at room temperature. Thaw these foods in a container on the bottom shelf of the refrigerator to keep juices from dripping on other foods.
- When barbecuing, precook meats just before putting them on the grill to make sure that the inside reaches the proper temperature.
- Eat meats and meat dishes while they are hot, and store leftovers in the refrigerator immediately. Don't let them sit at room temperature for more than 2 hours.

Eggs

- At the grocery store, make sure that egg shells are not cracked. Be sure to refrigerate eggs immediately after purchase and until you are ready to use them. Never let eggs or dishes prepared with eggs sit out at room temperature.
- Don't eat eggs that are soft-boiled, scrambled but runny, or sunny-side-up. Other foods prepared with uncooked or undercooked eggs—Caesar salad dressing, chocolate mousse, some frostings, homemade eggnog, and homemade mayonnaise—also should be avoided. If you eat home-made ice cream, check to see if raw eggs are an ingredient.
- If a recipe calls for raw eggs and the mixture will not be cooked, use a frozen egg product that has been pasteurized (heat treated for safety). This product will serve the same purpose as the raw eggs.

Milk and dairy products

- Buy only pasteurized milk and dairy products. Read the labels on cheeses; not all of them are pasteurized.
- Check the expiration date. Buy products before the expiration date on the package and use them within several days.
- Don't eat cheese that has mold on it.

Fruits and vegetables

- Choose fresh fruits and vegetables with unbroken skins.
- Wash thoroughly and peel raw fruits and vegetables with skin that may hide soil particles.
- Avoid moldy fruits and vegetables or produce with soft spots that show signs of mold.

Eating away from home

- Be sure your eating utensils, place settings, and beverage glasses are clean. Don't be shy about returning dirty utensils, food that is not hot enough, or food that is not cooked thoroughly.
- It may be best to avoid salad bars because you can't be sure how well the vegetables or fruits have been washed or how they have been handled. If you are given a choice between salad or soup, choose the soup.
- To be sure that meats are cooked thoroughly, order them medium-well to well-done.

From looking at this chapter, you might get the impression that just because you have HIV, eating becomes a big, complicated project. It doesn't. True, you may need to adjust what you eat depending on how you're feeling and to follow some basic food safety rules, but these changes are really not very difficult. Also, you can keep this book handy to look things up if you have questions.

But the most important nutrition rule is simple: Enjoy your food! Eating good food should always be a pleasure. With just a little thought and planning, mealtime can be one of the best parts of the day.

Refrigerated Products Stored at 35° to 40°F	Use Within
• Raw beefsteaks and roasts, raw pork chops, raw lamb chops and roasts, cooked ham, lunch meat	3–5 days
• Ground beef, turkey, pork, or lamb; sausage	1–2 days
• Hot dogs	1 week
• Raw chicken or turkey; giblets; raw fish	1–2 days
• Leftover cooked meat and meat dishes; soups and stews	3–4 days
• Leftover gravy and meat broth	1–2 days
• Leftover cooked poultry and poultry dishes	3–4 days
• Leftover cooked poultry covered with broth or gravy; leftover chicken nuggets, patties, or fried chicken	1–2 days
• Fresh eggs in the shell	3 weeks
• Raw yolks or whites (out of the shell)	2–4 days
• Hard-cooked eggs	1 week

PART

4

Managing
Health Care

10

Communicating

"Y*ou just don't understand!*" How often has this statement, expressed or unexpressed, summed up a frustrating verbal exchange? The goal in any communication between people is, first, that the other person understand what you are trying to say. Feeling you are not understood leads to frustration, and a prolonged feeling of frustration can lead to depression, anger, and helplessness. These are not good feelings for anyone, especially people with chronic illness. Dealing with a chronic illness can be frustrating enough without adding communication problems.

Poor communication is the biggest factor in poor relationships, whether they be between spouses, other family members or friends, coworkers, or doctors and patients. Even in casual relationships, poor communication causes frustration. How often have you been angry and frustrated as a customer, and how often is this because of poor communication?

When you have a chronic illness, good communication becomes a necessity. Your health care team, in particular, *must* "understand" you. As a self-manager, it is in your best interest to learn the skills necessary to make the communications in your life the most effective possible. In this chapter, we discuss ways to improve the communication process: how to express feelings in a positive way, how to ask for help, how to say "no," how to listen, and how to get more information from the other person.

While reading this chapter, keep in mind that *communication is a two-way street*. As uncomfortable as you may feel about expressing your feelings and asking for help, chances are that others are also feeling this way. It may be up to you to make sure the lines of communication are open.

Verbalizing Feelings—"I" Messages

Let's face it, many of us are uncomfortable expressing our feelings. Discomfort can be acute if doing so means we might seem critical of the person we're talking to. Especially if emotions are high, attempts to express frustration can be laden with *"you" messages. You* can be an accusatory word, suggesting blame. Its direction is toward the other person. Its use, when expressing feelings, can cause the other person to feel as though he or she is under attack. Suddenly, the other person feels on the defensive, and protective barriers go up. The person trying to express feelings, in turn, feels greater anxiety when faced with these defensive barriers, and the situation escalates to anger, frustration, and bad feelings.

I, on the other hand, is not an accusatory word. It doesn't strike out or blame. When expressing your own feelings, express them in terms of how *you* feel, not how the other person *makes* you feel.

The following are some examples of *"I" messages:*

"You" message:	"Why are *you* always late? We never get anywhere on time."
"I" message:	"*I* get really upset when *I'm* late. It's important to *me* to be on time."
"You" message:	"There's no way *you* can understand how lousy I feel."
"I" message:	"*I'm* not feeling well. *I* could really use a little help today."

Watch out for *hidden* "you" messages that are "you" messages with *"I feel* . . ."* stuck in front of them:

"You" message:	"*You* always walk too fast."
Hidden "you" message:	"*I feel* angry when *you* walk so fast."
"I" message:	"*I* have a hard time walking fast."

The trick to "I" messages is to avoid the use of the word *you* and to instead report your personal feelings using the word *I*. Of course, like any new skill, "I" messages take practice. Start by really listening, both to yourself and to others. Take some of the "you" messages you hear and turn them into "I" messages in your head. By playing this little word game in your head, you'll be surprised at how fast "I" messages become a habit in your own expressions.

There are some cautions to note when using "I" messages. First, they are

"I" Messages Exercise

Change the following statements into "I" messages. (Watch out for hidden "you" messages!) When you have finished the exercise, compare your "I" messages with our suggestions at the bottom of the page.

(1) You expect me to wait on you hand and foot!

(2) Doctor, you never have enough time for me. You're always in a hurry.

(3) You hardly ever touch me anymore. You don't pay any attention to me since my heart attack.

(4) You don't tell me the side effects of all these drugs you're giving me or why I have to take them, doctor.

not a miracle cure. Sometimes the listener has to have time to hear them. This is especially true if "you" messages and blaming have been the more usual ways of communicating. Even if at first using "I" messages seems ineffective, continue to use them and refine your skill. Some people may use "I" messages as a means of manipulation. If used in this way, problems can escalate. To be used effectively, "I" messages must report *honest* feelings.

Note: "I" messages are an excellent way to express *positive* feelings and compliments! "I really appreciate the extra time you gave me today, doctor."

Asking for Help

Problems with communication around the subject of help are pretty common. For some reason, many people feel awkward about asking for help or in refusing help. Although this problem is probably universal, it can come up more often for people with chronic illness.

Sample answers to "I" Messages Exercise, above:

(1) I'm frustrated by your illness. I feel as though I'm doing more than my share right now.

(2) Doctor, there doesn't seem to be enough time during our visits to address my concerns. I really feel rushed.

(3) I'm concerned that we seem to have grown apart since my heart attack.

(4) I don't feel well informed about the drugs I'm taking, doctor. *Or:* I feel I need to understand more about the medications I'm taking.

It may be emotionally difficult for some of us to ask for needed help. Maybe it's difficult for us to admit to ourselves that we are unable to do things as easily as in the past. When this is the case, try to avoid hedging your request with: "I'm sorry to have to ask this . . . ," "I know this is asking a lot . . . ," "I hate to ask this, but . . ." Hedging tends to put the other person on the defensive: "Gosh, what's he going to ask for that's so much, anyway?" Be specific about what help you are requesting. A general request can lead to misunderstanding, and the other person can react negatively to insufficient information.

General request:	"I know this is the last thing you want to do, but I need help moving. Will you help me?"
Reaction:	"Uh . . . well . . . I don't know. Um . . . can I get back to you after I check my schedule?" (Probably next year!)
Specific request:	"I'm moving next week, and I'd like to move my books and kitchen stuff ahead of time. Would you mind helping me load and unload the boxes in my car Saturday morning? I think it can be done in one trip."
Reaction:	"I'm busy Saturday morning, but I could give you a hand Friday night, if you'd like."

People with chronic illness must also sometimes deal with offers of help that are not needed nor desired. In most cases, these offers come from people who are dear to you and genuinely want to be helpful. A well-worded "I" message can refuse the help tactfully, without embarrassing the other person: "Thank you for being so thoughtful, but today I think I can handle it myself. I'd like to be able to take you up on your offer another time, though!"

Saying No

Suppose, however, you are the one being asked to help someone? Responding with yes or no may not be readily advisable. Often we need more information before we can respond to the request. If the request lacks enough information for us to respond, often our first reaction to the request is negative. The example we just discussed about helping a person move is a good one. "Help me move" can mean anything from moving furniture up stairs to picking up the pizza for the hungry troops. Again, using skills that get at the specifics will aid the communication process. It is important to understand what the *specific* request is before responding. *Asking for more information* or *paraphrasing* the request will often help clarify it, especially if prefaced by a phrase such as "Before I answer . . ." (this will hopefully prevent the person that you are paraphrasing from thinking that you are going to say yes).

Once you know what the specific request is and have decided to decline, it is important to *acknowledge the importance of the request* to the other person. In this way, the person will see that you are rejecting the *request*, rather than the *person*. Your turn-down should not be a put-down. "You know, that's a worthwhile project you're doing, but I think it's beyond my capabilities this week." Again, specifics are the key. Try to be clear about the conditions of your turn-down. Will you always turn down this request, or is it just that today or this week or right now is a problem?

Listening

Listening is probably the most important communication skill. Most of us are much better at talking than we are at listening. You need to actually listen to what the other person is *saying and feeling*. Most of us are already preparing a response instead of just listening.

There are several levels involved in being a good listener:

1. *Listen to the words and tone of voice, and observe body language.* Sometimes it is difficult to begin a conversation if there is a problem. There may be times when the words a person is saying don't tell you there is something bothering this person. Is the voice wavering? Does he or she appear to be struggling to find "the right words"? Do you notice body tension? Does he or she seem distracted? If you pick up on some of these signs, this person probably has more on his or her mind than words are expressing.

2. *Acknowledge having heard the other person.* Let the person know you heard them. This may be a simple "uh huh." Many times the only thing the other person wants is acknowledgment, or just someone to listen, because sometimes merely talking to a sympathetic listener is helpful.

3. *Acknowledge the content of the problem.* Let the other person know you heard the content and emotional level of the problem. You can do this by restating what you heard. For example, the content: "You are planning a trip." Or you can respond by acknowledging the emotions: "That must be difficult," or "You seem sad about it." When you respond on an emotional level,

the results are often startling. These responses tend to open the gates for more expression of feelings and thoughts. Responding to either the content or emotion can help communication along by discouraging the other person from repeating himself or herself, too.

4. *Respond by seeking more information.* This is especially important if you are not completely clear about what is being said or what is wanted. There is more than one useful method for seeking and getting information.

Getting More Information

Getting more information from another person is a bit of an art. Some of these methods are simple, others more subtle.

Ask for More

Asking is the simplest way to get more information. "Tell me more" will probably get you more, as will "I don't understand . . . please explain," "I would like to know more about . . . ," "Would you say that another way?" "How do you mean?" "I'm not sure I got that," and "Could you expand on that?"

Paraphrase

Paraphrasing is a good tool if you want to make sure you understand what the other person meant (not just what he or she *said*, but what was *meant*). Paraphrasing can either help or hinder effective communication, depending on the way the paraphrase is worded, though. It is important to remember to paraphrase in the form of a *question*, not a statement:

Original statement:	"Well, I don't know. I'm really not feeling up to par. This party will be crowded, there'll probably be smokers there, and I really don't know the hosts very well, anyway."
(1) *Paraphrased as a statement:*	"Obviously, you're telling me you don't want to go to the party."
(2) *Paraphrased as a question:*	"Are you saying that you'd rather stay home than go to the party?"

The response to the first paraphrase might be anger:

"No, I didn't say that! If you're going to be that way, I'll stay home
for sure."

Or, the response might be no response . . . a total shutdown of the communication, either because of anger or despair ("He just doesn't understand").
People don't like to be told what they meant.

The response to the second paraphrase might be more openness:

"That's not what I meant. I'm just feeling a little nervous about meeting
new people. I'd appreciate it if you'd stay near me during the party. I'd
feel better about it and I might have a good time."

As you can see, the second paraphrase promotes further communication, and
you have discovered the real reason the person was expressing doubt about
the party. You have gotten more information from the second paraphrase (the
question) and no new information from the first one (the statement).

Be Specific

If you want specific information, you must ask specific questions. We often
automatically speak in generalities:

Doctor: How have you been feeling?

Patient: Not so good.

The doctor's question doesn't produce much in the way of information about
the patient's condition. "Not so good" isn't very useful. Here's how the doctor
gets more information:

Doctor: Are you still having those sharp pains in your left arm?

Patient: Yes. A lot.

Doctor: How often?

Patient: A couple of times a day.

Doctor: How long do they last?

Patient: A long time.

Doctor: About how many minutes, would you say?

. . . and so on. Physicians have been trained in ways to get specific information from patients, but most of us have not been trained to ask specific
questions. Again, simply *asking for specifics* often works: "Can you be more specific about . . . ?" "Are you thinking of something particular?" If you want to
know "why," be specific about what it is. If you ask a specific question, you will
be more likely to get a specific answer.

Simply asking *"Why?"* can unnecessarily prolong your attempt to get specific information from the doctor. In addition to being a general rather than a specific word, *why* also makes a person think in terms of cause and effect, and he or she may respond at an entirely different level than you had in mind. Most of us have experienced a three-year-old who just keeps asking "Why?" over and over and over again until the information he or she wants is finally obtained (or the parent runs from the room, screaming). The poor parent doesn't have the faintest idea what the child has in mind, and answers "Because . . ." in an increasingly specific order until the child's question is answered. Sometimes, however, the direction the answers take is entirely different than the child's question, and the child never gets the information he or she wanted. Rather than *why*, begin your questions with *who, which, when, where,* or *what.* These words promote a specific response. For example:

Doctor:	I'm going to send you for a colonoscopy.
Patient:	Why?
Doctor:	Well, because I feel that anyone with blood in his stool should have one.
Patient:	Why is that?
Doctor:	It's medically indicated.

. . . and so on. This questioning could go on for a long time, and the patient's question "Why?" may hide any number of different concerns. Compare the conversation above with this one:

Doctor:	I'm going to send you for a colonoscopy.
Patient:	What do you think might be wrong?
Doctor:	I'm not sure. It's probably not serious, but you could have a cancer, like lymphoma.
Patient:	Who does the colonoscopy? You?
Doctor:	No, Dr. Jones, the GI specialist, will do it.

. . . and so on. Asking specific questions like these helps you communicate better and helps avoid misunderstandings.

Communicating with Your Doctor

As a person with chronic illness, it is especially important for you to establish and maintain good communications with your doctor. The relationship you have with him or her must be looked on as a long-term one requiring regular work, much like a business partnership or a marriage. Your doctor will probably know more intimate details about you than anyone except perhaps your spouse, partner, or parents. You, in turn, should feel comfortable expressing your fears, asking questions that you may think are "stupid," and negotiating a treatment plan to satisfy both you and your doctor without feeling "put down" or that your doctor is not interested.

There are two things to keep in mind that will help open, and keep open, the lines of communication with your doctor. First, *how does the doctor feel?* Too often, we expect our doctor to act like a warm-hearted computer—a gigantic brain stuffed with knowledge about the human body, able to analyze the situation and produce a diagnosis, prognosis, and treatment on demand— *and* be a warm, caring person who makes us feel as though we are the only person he or she cares about taking care of. Actually, most doctors wish they were just that sort of person, but no doctor can be all things to all patients. They are human, too. They get headaches, they get tired, and they get sore feet. They have families who demand their time and attention, and they have to fight bureaucracies as formidable as the rest of us face.

Most doctors entered the grueling medical training system because they wanted to make sick people well. It is frustrating for them not to be able to cure someone with a disease like HIV/AIDS. They must take their satisfaction in their chosen profession in improvements rather than cures, or even in maintenance of existing conditions rather than declines. Undoubtedly, you have been frustrated, angry, or depressed from time to time about your illness, but bear in mind that your doctor has probably felt similar emotions about his or her inability to make you well. In this, you are truly partners.

Second, in this partnership between you and your doctor, *the biggest threat to a good relationship and good communication is time.* If you or your doctor could have a fantasy about the best thing to happen in your relationship, it would probably involve more time for you both, more time to discuss things, more time to explain things, more time to explore options. When time is short, the anxiety it produces can bring about rushed messages—often "you" messages, and messages that are just plain misunderstood—with no time to correct them.

A doctor is usually on a very tight schedule. This fact becomes painfully obvious to you when you have had to wait in the doctor's office because an emergency has happened at some time before an appointment. Doctors try to stay on schedule, and sometimes patients and doctors alike feel rushed as a consequence. One way to help you to get the most from your visit with the doctor is to take **"PART"**:

Prepare. Ask. Repeat. Take action.

Prepare

Before visiting or calling your doctor, *prepare your "agenda."* What are the reasons for your visit? What do you expect from your doctor? Take some time to make a written list of your concerns or questions. But be realistic. If you have thirteen different problems, it isn't likely that your doctor can adequately deal with that many concerns in one visit. Identify your *main* concerns or problems. Writing them down also helps you remember them. Have you ever thought to yourself, after you walked out of the doctor's office, "Why didn't I ask about . . ." or "I forgot to mention . . ." Making a list beforehand helps ensure that your main concerns get addressed.

Preparing will also help you to do several important things *during* the visit.

- *Mention your main concerns right at the beginning of the visit.* Don't wait until the end of the appointment to bring up concerns, because there won't be the time to properly deal with them. Give your list to the doctor. Make the list in order of the importance of your concerns, and let your doctor know which items are the most important to you. If the list is long, expect that only two or three items will be addressed this visit. Studies show that doctors allow an average of eighteen seconds for the patient to state his or her concerns before interrupting with focused questioning. Preparing your questions in advance will help you use your eighteen seconds well. Remember to check your list before you leave the appointment to make sure your most important concerns have been addressed.

- As an example of bringing up your major concerns at the beginning of the visit, when the doctor asks, "What brings you in today?" you might say something like, "I have a lot of things I want to discuss this visit" *(the doctor immediately begins to feel anxious because of an already overfull appointment schedule),* "but I know that we have a limited amount of time. The things that most concern me are my shoulder pain, my dizziness, and the side effects from one of the medications I'm taking" *(the doctor feels relieved because the concerns are focused and potentially manageable within the appointment time available).*

- *Try to be as open as you can in sharing your thoughts, feelings, and fears.* Remember, your physician is not a mind reader. If you are worried, try to explain *why.* "I am worried that what I have may be contagious," or

"My father had similar symptoms before he died," and so on. The more open you are, the more likely it is that your doctor can help you.

- *Give your physician feedback.* If you don't like the way you have been treated by the physician or someone else on the health care team, let your physician know. If you were unable to follow the physician's advice or had problems with a treatment, tell your physician so adjustments can be made. Also, most physicians appreciate compliments and positive feedback, but patients are often hesitant to praise their doctors. So if you are pleased, remember to let your physician know this, too.

- *Be prepared to concisely describe your symptoms to the doctor:* when they started; how long they last; where they are located; what makes them better or worse; whether you have had similar problems before; whether you have changed your diet, exercise, or medications in a way that might contribute to the symptoms; and so on. If a treatment has been tried, you should be prepared to report the effect of the treatment. And if you have previous records or test results that might be relevant to your problems, bring them along.

Ask

Another key to effective doctor-patient communication is asking questions. Getting understandable answers and information is one of the cornerstones of self-management.

You need to be prepared to ask questions about diagnosis, tests, treatments, and follow-up.

- *Diagnosis.* Ask your doctor what's wrong, what caused it, if it is contagious, what the future outlook (or prognosis) is, and what can be done to prevent it in the future.

- *Tests.* Ask your doctor if any medical tests are necessary, how they will affect your treatment, how accurate they are, and what is likely to happen if you are not tested. If you decide to have a test, find out how to prepare for the test and what it will be like.

- *Treatments.* Ask about your treatment options, including lifestyle changes, medications, and surgery. Inquire about the risks and benefits of treatment and the consequences of not treating.

- *Follow-up.* Find out if and when you should call or return for a follow-up visit. What symptoms should you watch for, and what should you do if they occur?

You may wish to take some notes on important points during the visit or consider bringing along someone else to act as a second listener. Another set of eyes and ears may help you later recall some of the details of the visit or instruction.

Repeat

It is extremely helpful to briefly repeat back to the doctor some of the key points from the visit and discussion, such as diagnosis, prognosis, next steps, treatment actions, and so on. This is to double-check that you clearly understood the most important information. Repeating back also gives the doctor a chance to quickly correct any misunderstandings and miscommunications. If you don't understand or remember something the physician said, admit that you need to go over it again. For example, you might say, "I'm pretty sure you told me some of this before, but I'm still confused about it." Don't be afraid to ask what you may consider a "stupid" question. These questions can often indicate an important concern or misunderstanding.

Take Action

When the visit is ending, you need to clearly understand what to do next. When appropriate, ask your physician to write down instructions or recommend reading material for more information on a particular subject.

If, for some reason, you can't or won't follow the doctor's advice, let the doctor know. For example, "I can't take the aspirin. It gives me stomach problems," or "My insurance doesn't cover that much physical therapy, so I can't afford it," or "I've tried to exercise before, but I can't seem to keep it up." If your doctor knows why you can't or won't follow advice, he or she can sometimes make alternative suggestions to help you overcome the barrier. If you don't share the barriers to taking actions, it's difficult for your doctor to help.

Asking for a Second Opinion

Many people find it uncomfortable to ask their doctor for a second opinion about their diagnosis or treatment. Especially if you have a long relationship with your doctor or simply *like* him or her, you may sometimes worry that asking for another opinion might be interpreted as questioning the doctor's competence. It is a rare doctor whose feelings will be hurt by a sincere request for another opinion. If your condition is medically complicated or difficult, the doctor may have already consulted with another doctor (or more) about your case, at least on an informal basis.

Even if your condition is not particularly complicated, asking for a second opinion is a perfectly acceptable, and often expected, request. Doctors prefer a straightforward request, and asking in a nonthreatening "I" message will make this task simple:

"*I'm* still feeling confused and uncomfortable about this treatment.
I feel another opinion might help *me* feel more reassured. Can you suggest someone I could consult?"

In this way, you have expressed your own feelings without suggesting that the doctor is at fault. You have also confirmed your confidence in him or her by asking that he or she suggest the other doctor. (Remember, however, that you are not bound by his or her suggestion; you may choose anyone you wish for a second opinion.)

Good communication skills help make life easier for everyone, especially when chronic illness enters the picture. The skills discussed in this chapter, though brief, will hopefully help smooth the communication process. In summary, the following box gives some words that can help or hinder:

Words That Help	*Words That Hinder*
• "I"	• "You"
• Right now, at this time, at this point, today	• Never, always, every time, constantly
• Who, which, where, when	• Obviously . . .
• How do you mean, please explain, tell me more, I don't understand	• Why

Suggested Reading

Beck, Aaron T. *Love Is Never Enough: How Couples Can Overcome Misunderstandings, Resolve Conflicts, and Solve Relationship Problems Through Cognitive Therapy.* New York: Harper & Row, 1988. (A good introduction to cognitive techniques for couples.)

Golde, Robert A. *What You Say Is What You Get.* New York: Hawthorn Books, 1979.

McKay, Matthew, Martha Davis, and Patrick Fanning. Messages: The Communication Skills Book. Oakland, Calif.: New Harbinger Publications, 1983.

11

Making Your Wishes Known— Durable Power of Attorney for Health Care

All of us, whether ill or healthy, have feelings about our own death. Death may be feared, welcomed, accepted, or, all too often, pushed aside to be thought about at a different time. Somewhere, in the back of our minds, though, most of us have ideas about how and when we would like to die. For some of us, life is so important that we feel that everything should be done to sustain it. For others of us, life is important only so long as we can be active participants. For many people, the issue isn't really death but, rather, dying. We may have heard about the eighty-year-old who died skiing. This may be considered a "good" death. On the other hand, we may have a friend who spent a long time in a nursing home unaware of his or her surroundings. This is usually not what we would wish for ourselves.

Although none of us can have absolute control over our own death, this, like the rest of our life, is something we can help manage. That is, we can have input, make decisions, and probably add a great deal to the quality of our death. Proper management can lessen the negative impacts of our death on our survivors.

This chapter presents information that will help you better manage some of the legal issues of death, specifically the durable power of attorney for health care. Although each state has different regulations, the information presented here should be useful wherever you live. You can get information and forms specific for your state by writing to the Society for the Right to Die. The address is on page 158.

Durable Power of Attorney
for Health Care

A durable power of attorney for health care is a document that *appoints another person to act in your place if you are unable to do so*. It differs from a living will in two ways. First, a living will is good only in case of a terminal illness, whereas a durable power of attorney for health care can apply to any illness. Second, a durable power of attorney for health care allows you to appoint another person to act for you. A living will does not allow for this provision. For example, when parents go on trips, they often leave a friend or other family member with the power of attorney so that someone can take care of any emergency that might happen with the children. A durable power of attorney *for health care* is a document in which you appoint someone else to act for you, or act as your agent, concerning health care. In other words, it allows someone else to make decisions for you concerning your health care only. It does not give them the right to act for you in other ways, such as handling your financial matters. This document is activated only when for some reason you are unable to make decisions yourself (for example, if you are in a coma or become mentally incompetent).

Besides naming someone as your agent, the durable power of attorney can give *guidelines* to your agent about your *wishes concerning health care*. You do not have to give guidance to your agent. However, many people wish to do so. This guidance indicates almost anything you want done for your care; it may range from use of aggressive life-sustaining measures to the withholding of life-sustaining measures.

To complete a durable power of attorney for health care means making many decisions. To help you understand the decisions you will be asked to make we have included a sample of a form used in California at the end of this chapter. Each part of the following discussion is lettered. A similar letter appears at the appropriate points on the sample form. The headings in the discussion parallel the headings of the respective sections in the form.

A Designation of Health Care Agent

First, you must decide who you want to be your agent. The person can be a friend or family member. It cannot be the physician who is providing your care. There are some considerations to be made in choosing your agent. This person should generally be available in the geographic area where you live. If the agent is not available to make decisions for you, he or she is not much help. Just to be on the safe side, you can also name a backup agent who would act in your behalf if your primary agent was not available. Second, you must be sure that this person thinks like you think or at least would be willing to carry out your wishes. Third, the person must be someone who you feel would be able to carry out your wishes. Sometimes a partner or child is not the best agent because this person is too close to you emotionally. For example, if you wish not to be resuscitated in the case of a severe coma, your agent has to be able to tell the doctor not to resuscitate. This could be very difficult or impossible for a family member or partner to decide then and there. Be sure the person you choose as your agent is up to this task and would not say "Do everything you can" at this critical time. Finally, you want your agent to be someone who will not find this job too much of an emotional burden. Thus, the person has to be comfortable with the role, as well as willing and able to carry out your wishes.

In review, look for these characteristics in an agent:

- Someone who is likely to be available should he or she need to act on your behalf
- Someone who understands your wishes and is willing to carry them out
- Someone who is emotionally prepared and able to carry out your wishes
- Someone who will not be emotionally burdened by carrying out your wishes

As you can see, finding the right agent is a very important task. You may want to talk to several people before making your choice—these may be the most important interviews that you ever conduct. We will talk more about discussing your wishes with family, friends, and your doctor later.

B General Statement of Authority Granted

The other major decision you may want to make is what you want to put in your durable power of attorney for health care. In other words, what are your directions to your agent? Some forms make a "general statement of authority granted," in which you give your agent full power to make decisions. You do not write out the details of what these decisions should be—you are trusting your agent to follow your wishes. Since these wishes are not explicitly written, it is very important that you have discussed them in detail with your agent.

C Statement of Desires Concerning Medical Treatment

Some forms give you a choice of several general statements of desires concerning your medical treatment. All you need to do is to initial the statement that best applies to you.

> I do *not* want my life to be prolonged and I do *not* want life-sustaining treatment to be provided or continued: (1) if I am in an irreversible coma or persistent vegetative state; or (2) if I am terminally ill and the application of life-sustaining procedures would serve only to artificially delay the moment of my death; or (3) under any other circumstances where the burdens of the treatment outweigh the expected benefits. I want my agent to consider the relief of suffering and the quality as well as the extent or the possible extension of my life in making decisions concerning life-sustaining treatment.

> I want my life to be prolonged and I want life-sustaining treatment to be provided *unless I am in a coma or vegetative state* which my doctor reasonably believes to be irreversible. Once my doctor has reasonably concluded that I will remain unconscious for the rest of my life, I do *not* want life-sustaining treatment to be provided or continued.

> I want my life to be prolonged to the greatest extent possible without regard to my condition, the chances I have for recovery or the cost of the procedures.

D Other or Additional Statements of Desires, Special Provisions, or Limitations

All forms also have a space in which you can write out any specific wishes that either limit or add to the authority you have given your agent in the general statement you have initialed. You are not required to give specific details but may wish to do so. Knowing what details to write is a little complicated because you do not know the exact circumstances in which the agent will have to act. However, you can get some idea by asking your doctor about what he thinks might be the most likely things to happen to someone with your condition. Then you can direct your agent on how to act. Your specific directions can discuss outcomes, specific circumstances, or both. If you discuss outcomes, the statement should focus on what types of outcomes would be acceptable and which would not. For example, "Resuscitate if I can continue to fully function mentally."

The following are two of the more common specific circumstances that are encountered with HIV/AIDS:

- *AIDS dementia complex* is a disease that can leave you with little or no mental function. In spite of this, it is generally not life threatening, at least not for a long time. However, things happen to people with AIDS dementia complex that can be life-threatening, such as pneumonia, meningitis, and wasting. What you need to do is decide how much treatment you want. For example, do you want antibiotics if you get pneumonia? Do you want to be resuscitated if you die in your sleep? Do you wish a feeding tube if you are unable to feed yourself? Remember, it is your choice as to how you answer each of these questions. You may not want to be resuscitated, but may want a feeding tube. If you want aggressive treatment, you may want to use all means to sustain life or, more conservatively, you may not want any special means used to sustain life. For example, you may want to be fed but may not want to be placed on life support equipment.

- You may have a *very bad lung function* that will not improve. Should you be unable to breathe on your own, do you want to be placed in an intensive care unit on mechanical ventilation (a breathing machine)? Remember, this is a situation in which you will not improve. To say that you never want ventilation is very different from saying that you don't want it if it is used to sustain life when no improvement is likely. Obviously, mechanical ventilation can be life-saving in such crises as a severe asthma attack, when it is used for a short time until the body can regain its normal function. Here, the issue is not whether to use mechanical ventilation ever, but rather when or under what circumstances you wish it be used.

These examples may give you some ideas regarding the directions you would like to give in your durable power of attorney for health care. Again, to better understand how to write such directions, or how to make them more personal to your own condition, you might want to talk with your physician about what the common problems and decisions are for people like you.

In summary, there are several decisions you need to make in directing your agent on how to act in your behalf:

- Generally, *how much treatment do you want?* This can range from the very aggressive—that is, doing many things to sustain life—to the very conservative, which is doing almost nothing to sustain life, except to keep you clean and comfortable.

- Given the types of life-threatening things that are likely to happen to people with your condition, *what sorts of treatment do you want and under what conditions?*

- If you become *mentally incapacitated*, what sorts of treatment do you want for *other illnesses*, such as pneumonia?

Many people get this far. That is, they have thought through their wishes about dying and have even written them down in a durable power of attorney for health care. This is an excellent beginning, but not the end of the job. A good manager has to do more than just write a memo. He or she has to see that the memo gets delivered. If you really want your wishes carried out, it is important that you share them fully with your agent, your family, and your doctor. This is often not an easy task. In the following section, we will discuss ways to make these conversations easier.

Talking with Your Family, Friends, and Agent

E Before you can talk about your wishes with family, friends, and agent, all interested parties need to have copies of your durable power of attorney for health care. Once you have completed the documents, have them witnessed and signed. You can have your durable power of attorney notarized instead of having it witnessed. Make several copies at any copy center. You will need copies for your agent, family members, and your doctor. You may also want to give one to your lawyer.

Now you are ready to talk about your wishes. Nobody likes to discuss his or her own death or that of a loved one. Therefore, it is not surprising that when you bring up this subject the response is often "Oh, don't think about that," or "That's a long time off," or "Don't be so morbid, you're not that sick." Unfortunately, this is usually enough to end the conversation. Your job as a good self-manager is to keep the conversation open. Here are some suggestions on how to begin your discussion of this subject:

- *Prepare your durable power of attorney*, and then *give copies* to the appropriate family members or friends. *Ask them to read it* and then set a specific time to *discuss it*. If they give you one of those responses mentioned above, say that you understand this is a difficult topic, but that it is important to you that you discuss it with them. This is a good time to practice the "I" messages discussed in Chapter 11. For example, "I understand that death is a difficult thing to talk about. However, it is very important to me that we have this discussion."

- You might get *blank copies* of the durable power of attorney forms for all your family members and suggest that *you all fill them out and share them*. Present this task as an important aspect of being a mature adult and family member. Making this a family project in which everyone is involved may make it easier to discuss. Besides, it will help to clarify everyone's values about the topics of death and dying.

- If these two suggestions seem too difficult, or, for some reason, are impossible to carry out, you might *write a letter* or prepare an *audiotape* to send to members of your family. In the letter or tape, talk about why you feel your death is an important topic to discuss and that you want them to know your wishes. Then state your wishes, providing reasons for the choices you indicate. At the same time, send them a copy of your durable power of attorney for health care. Ask that they respond in some way, or perhaps you can set aside some time to talk with them in person or on the phone.

In deciding on your agent, it is important that you choose someone with whom you can talk freely and exchange ideas. If your chosen agent is not willing to or is unable to talk to you about your wishes, you have probably chosen the wrong person. Also, don't be fooled. Just because someone is very close does not mean that he or she really understands your wishes or would be able to carry them out. This is not a topic that should be left to a mutual, unspoken understanding unless you don't mind if your agent decides differently from what you wish. For this reason, choosing someone who is not close to you emotionally is sometimes better. Talking with your agent is especially important if you have not written details of your wishes.

Talking with Your Doctor

From our research we have learned that, in general, people have a much more difficult time talking to their doctors about their wishes surrounding death than to their families. In fact, only a very small percentage of people who have written durable powers of attorney for health care ever share these with their physician. There are several reasons why it is important that such a discussion take place. First, you need to *be sure that your doctor has values that are compatible with your wishes*. If you and your doctor do not have the same values, it may be difficult for him or her to carry out your wishes. Second, *your doctor needs to know what you want*. This allows him or her to take appropriate actions, such as writing orders to resuscitate or not to use mechanical resuscitation should this be needed. Third, *your doctor needs to know who your agent is and how to contact this person.* If an important decision has to be made and your wishes are to be followed, the doctor must talk with your agent. It is important to give your doctor a copy of your durable power of attorney for health care, so that it can become a permanent part of your medical record. Again, the problem is often how you start this conversation with your doctor.

As surprising as it may seem, many physicians also find it difficult to discuss death and how it might occur with their patients. After all they are in the business of helping to keep people alive and well. They don't like to think about their patients dying. On the other hand, most doctors want their patients to have durable powers of attorney for health care. This relieves them of pressure and worry.

If you wish, *plan a time with your doctor when you can discuss your wishes.* This should not be a side conversation at the end of a regular visit. Rather, start a visit by saying, "I want a few minutes to discuss with you my wishes in the event of a serious problem or impending death." When you put it this way, most doctors will make time to talk with you. If the doctor says that he or she does not have enough time, then ask when you can make another appointment to talk with him or her. This is a situation in which you may need to be a little assertive. Sometimes a doctor, like your family members or friends, might say "Oh, you don't have to worry about that, let me do it," or "We'll worry about that when the time comes." Again, you will have to take the initiative, using an "I" message to communicate that this is important to you and that you do not want to put off the discussion.

Sometimes doctors do not want to worry you. They think they are doing you a favor by not describing all the unpleasant things that might happen to you, or the potential treatments, in the case of serious problems. You can help your doctor by telling him or her that having control and making some decisions about your future will ease your mind. Not knowing or not being clear on what will happen is more worrisome than being faced with the facts, unpleasant as they may be, and dealing with them.

Even knowing all of the above, it is still sometimes hard to talk with your doctor. Therefore, it might also be helpful to *bring your agent with you* when you have this discussion. The agent can facilitate the discussion and, at the same time, meet your doctor. Having your agent present also gives everyone a chance to clarify any misunderstandings about your wishes. It opens the lines of communication so that if your agent and physician have to act to carry out your wishes, they can do so with few problems.

So now you have done all the important things. You can rest easy. The hard work is over. However, remember that you can change your mind at any time. Your agent may no longer be available or your wishes might change. Be sure to keep your durable power of attorney for health care updated. Like any legal document, it can be revoked or changed at any time. In all cases, it *must be updated every seven years*. However, if you are incapacitated when your durable power of attorney for health care expires, it will remain in effect until you can renew it. The decisions you make today are not forever.

One last note: Many states recognize durable powers of attorney for health care that are created in another state. However, this is not always the case. As of 1996, this is an unclear legal issue. To be on the safe side, if you move or spend a lot of time in another state, it is best to check with a lawyer in that state to see if your document is legally binding there.

Making your wishes known about how you want to be treated in case of serious or life-threatening illness is one of the most important tasks of self-management. The best way to do this is to prepare a durable power of attorney for health care and to share it with your family, important friends, and physician.

On the following pages, we show a sample durable power of attorney for health care developed for use in California. Be sure to check on the appropriate forms for your state by asking your doctor or lawyer or by writing to the Society for the Right to Die (see below).

Resources

Making Your Wishes Known

The Society for the Right to Die
250 West 57th Street, Room #323
New York, NY 10107

CALIFORNIA MEDICAL ASSOCIATION
DURABLE POWER OF ATTORNEY FOR HEALTH CARE FORM
INSTRUCTIONS AND CHECKLIST

This is a Durable Power of Attorney for Health Care form. By filling in this form, you can select someone to make health care decisions for you if for some reason you become unable to make those decisions for yourself. You can also specify any wishes you may have about your health care, including your desires concerning decisions to withhold or remove life-sustaining treatment. A properly completed form provides the best legal protection available to help ensure that your wishes will be respected.

READ THIS FORM CAREFULLY BEFORE FILLING IT OUT. EACH PARAGRAPH IN THE FORM CONTAINS IN-STRUCTIONS. IT IS IMPORTANT THAT YOU FOLLOW THESE INSTRUCTIONS SO THAT YOUR WISHES MAY BE CARRIED OUT.

The following checklist is provided to help you complete this form completely. If you have properly completed the form, you should be able to answer *yes* to each of the following:

_____ 1. I am a California resident who is at least 18 years old, of sound mind and acting of my own free will.

_____ 2. The individuals I have selected as my agent and alternate agents to make health care decisions for me are at least 18 years old and are *not:*
   - my *treating* health care provider.
   - an employee of my *treating* health care provider, unless the employee is related to me by blood, marriage or adoption.
   - an operator of a community care facility or residential care facility for the elderly. (Community care facilities are sometimes called board and care homes. If you are unsure whether a person you are thinking of selecting operates a community care facility, you should ask that person.)
   - an employee of a community care facility or residential care facility for the elderly, unless the employee is related to me by blood, marriage or adoption.

_____ 3. I have talked with the individuals I have selected as my agent and alternate agents and these individuals have agreed to participate. (You may select someone who is not a California resident to act as your agent or alternate agent, but you should consider whether someone who lives far away will be available to make decisions for you if and when that may become necessary.)

_____ 4. I have read the instructions and completed paragraphs 2, 4, 5, 6, 7, 8, and 9 to reflect my desires.

_____ 5. I have *signed* and *dated* the form.

_____ 6. I have either ____ had the form notarized; *or* ____ had the form properly witnessed:
   ___ a) I have obtained the signatures of two adult witnesses who personally know me.
   ___ b) Neither witness is: (1) my agent or alternate agent designated in this form; (2) a health care provider, or the employee of a health care provider; (3) a person who operates or is employed by a community care facility or residential care facility for the elderly.
   ___ c) At least one witness is not related to me by blood, marriage, or adoption, and is not named in my will or so far as I know entitled to any part of my estate when I die.

_____ 7. **I have given a copy of the completed form to those people, including my agent, alternate agents, family members, and doctor, who may need this form in case an emergency requires a decision concerning my health care.**

SPECIAL REQUIREMENTS

_____ 8. **Patients in Skilled Nursing Facilities:** If I am a patient in a skilled nursing facility, I have obtained the signature of a patient advocate or ombudsman. (If you are not sure whether you are in a skilled nursing facility, you should ask the people taking care of you.)

_____ 9. **Conservatees under the Lanterman-Petris-Short Act:** If I am a conservatee under the Lanterman-Petris-Short Act and want to select my conservator as my agent or alternate agent to make health care decisions, I have obtained a lawyer's certification. (If you are not sure whether the person you wish to select as your agent is your conservator under the Lanterman-Petris-Short Act, you should ask that person.)

If you change your mind about who you would like to make health care decisions for you, or about any of the other statements you have made in this form you should take all of the following steps: 1. Complete a new form with the changes you desire; 2. Tell everyone who got a copy of the old form that it is no longer valid and ask that copies of the old form be returned to you so you may destroy them; 3. Give copies of the new form to the people who may need the form to carry out your wishes as described above in number 7. If after reading this material you still have unanswered questions, you should talk to your doctor or a lawyer.

DURABLE POWER OF ATTORNEY FOR HEALTH CARE DECISIONS

(California Civil Code Sections 2410-2443)

WARNING TO PERSON EXECUTING THIS DOCUMENT

This is an important legal document. Before executing this document, you should know these important facts:

This document gives the person you designate as your agent (the attorney-in-fact) the power to make health care decisions for you. Your agent must act consistently with your desires as stated in this document or otherwise made known.

Except as you otherwise specify in this document, this document gives your agent power to consent to your doctor not giving treatment or stopping treatment necessary to keep you alive.

Notwithstanding this document, you have the right to make medical and other health care decisions for yourself so long as you can give informed consent with respect to the particular decision. In addition, no treatment may be given to you over your objection, and health care necessary to keep you alive may not be stopped or withheld if you object at the time.

This document gives your agent authority to consent, to refuse to consent, or to withdraw consent to any care, treatment, service, or procedure to maintain, diagnose, or treat a physical or mental condition. This power is subject to any statement of your desires and any limitations that you include in this document. You may state in this document any types of treatment that you do not desire. In addition, a court can take away the power of your agent to make health care decisions for you if your agent (1) authorizes anything that is illegal, (2) acts contrary to your known desires or (3) where your desires are not known, does anything that is clearly contrary to your best interests.

Unless you specify a shorter period in this document, this power will exist for seven years from the date you execute this document and, if you are unable to make health care decisions for yourself at the time when this seven-year period ends, this power will continue to exist until the time you become able to make health care decisions for yourself.

You have the right to revoke the authority of your agent by notifying your agent or your treating doctor, hospital, or other health care provider orally or in writing of the revocation.

Your agent has the right to examine your medical records and to consent to their disclosure unless you limit this right in this document.

Unless you otherwise specify in this document, this document gives your agent the power after you die to (1) authorize an autopsy, (2) donate your body or parts thereof for transplant or therapeutic or educational or scientific purposes, and (3) direct the disposition of your remains.

It there is anything in this document that you do not understand, you should ask a lawyer to explain it to you.

TERMS OF DURABLE POWER OF ATTORNEY FOR HEALTH CARE

1. CREATION OF DURABLE POWER OF ATTORNEY FOR HEALTH CARE

By this document I intend to create a durable power of attorney by appointing the person designated below to make health care decisions for me as allowed by Sections 2410 to 2443, inclusive, of the California Civil Code. This power of attorney shall not be affected by my subsequent incapacity.

A

2. DESIGNATION OF HEALTH CARE AGENT

(Insert the name and address of the person you wish to designate as your agent to make health care decisions for you. None of the following may be designated as your agent: (1) your treating health care provider, (2) a nonrelative employee of your treating health care provider, (3) an operator of a community care facility or residential care facility for the elderly, or (4) a nonrelative employee of an operator of a community care facility or residential care facility for the elderly.)

I, _____ **EXAMPLE** _____
(insert your name)

do hereby designate and appoint: _____
(name)

as my attorney-in-fact (agent) to make health care decisions for me as authorized in this document.

Address: _____

Telephone Number: _____

B 3. GENERAL STATEMENT OF AUTHORITY GRANTED

If I become incapable of giving informed consent to health care decisions, I hereby grant to my agent full power and authority to make health care decisions for me including the right to consent, refuse consent, or withdraw consent to any care, treatment, service, or procedure to maintain, diagnose or treat a physical or mental condition, and to receive and to consent to the release of medical information, subject to the statement of desires, special provisions and limitations set out in paragraph 4.

C 4. STATEMENT OF DESIRES CONCERNING MEDICAL TREATMENT

(Your agent must make health care decisions that are consistent with your known desires. You can, but are not required to, state your desires in the space provided below. You should consider whether you want to include a statement of your desires concerning decisions to withhold or remove life-sustaining treatment. For your convenience, some general statements concerning the withholding and removal of life-sustaining treatment are set out below. If you agree with one of these statements, you may INITIAL that statement. READ ALL OF THESE STATEMENTS CAREFULLY BEFORE YOU SELECT ONE TO INITIAL. You can also write your own statement concerning life-sustaining and/or other matters relating to your health care. BY LAW, YOUR AGENT IS NOT PERMITTED TO CONSENT ON YOUR BEHALF TO ANY OF THE FOLLOWING: COMMITMENT TO OR PLACEMENT IN A MENTAL HEALTH TREATMENT FACILITY, CONVULSIVE TREATMENT, PSYCHOSURGERY, STERILIZATION OR ABORTION. In every other respect, your agent may make health care decisions for you to the same extent you could make them for yourself if you were capable of doing so. If you want to limit in any other way the authority given your agent by this document, you should state the limits in the space below. If you do not initial one of the printed statements or write your own statement, your agent will have the broad powers to make health care decisions on your behalf which are set forth in Paragraph 3, except to the extent that there are limits provided by law.)

I do **not** want my life to be prolonged and I do **not** want life-sustaining treatment to be provided or continued: (1) if I am in an irreversible coma or persistent vegetative state; or (2) if I am terminally ill and the application of life sustaining procedures would serve only to artificially delay the moment of my death; or (3) under any other circumstances where the burdens of the treatment outweigh the expected benefits. I want my agent to consider the relief of suffering and the quality as well as the extent of the possible extension of my life in making decisions concerning life-sustaining treatment.

If this statement reflects your desires initial here: ____ **EXAMPLE** ____

I want my life to be prolonged and I want life sustaining treatment to be provided **unless I am in a coma or vegetative state** which my doctor reasonably believes to be irreversible. Once my doctor has reasonably concluded that I will remain unconscious for the rest of my life, I do **not** want life-sustaining treatment to be provided or continued.

If this statement reflects your desires initial here: ____ **EXAMPLE** ____

I want my life to be prolonged to the greatest extent possible without regard to my condition, the chances I have for recovery or the cost of the procedures.

If this statement reflects your desires initial here: ____ **EXAMPLE** ____

D Other or additional statements of desires, special provisions, or limitations:

_____

_____

_____ EXAMPLE _____

_____

_____

_____

(You may attach additional pages if you need more space to complete your statement. If you attach additional pages, you must DATE and SIGN EACH PAGE.)

161

E **5. DESIGNATION OF ALTERNATE AGENTS**

(You are not required to designate any alternate agents but you may do so. Any alternative agent you designate will be able to make the same health care decisions as the agent designated in Paragraph 2, above, in the event that agent is unable or unwilling to act as your agent. Also, if the agent designated in Paragraph 2 is your spouse, his or her designation as your agent is automatically revoked by law if your marriage is dissolved.)

If the person designated in Paragraph 2 as my agent is not available and willing to make a health care decision for me, then I designate the following persons to serve as my agent to make health care decisions for me as authorized in this document, such persons to serve in the order listed below:

A. First Alternative Agent

 Name: _____

 Address: _____

 Telephone:_____

B. Second Alternative Agent

 Name: _____

 Address: _____

 Telephone:_____

6. DURATION

I understand that this power of attorney will exist for seven years from the date I execute this document unless I establish a shorter time. If I am unable to make health care decisions for myself when this power of attorney expires, the authority I have granted my agent will continue to exist until the time when I become able to make health care decisions for myself.

(Optional) I wish to have this power of attorney end before seven years on the following date: _____. (Fill in this space ONLY if you want the authority of your agent to end EARLIER than the seven-year period described above.)

7. NOMINATION OF CONSERVATOR OF MY PERSON

(A conservator of the person may be appointed for you if a court decides that you are unable properly to provide for your personal needs for physical health, food, clothing, or shelter. The appointment of a conservator may affect, or transfer to the conservator, your right to control your physical care, including under some circumstances your right to make health care decisions. You are not required to nominate a conservator but you may do so. The court will appoint the person you nominate unless that would be contrary to your best interests. You may, but are not required to, nominate as your conservator the same person you named in paragraph 2 as your health care agent. You can nominate an individual as your conservator by completing the space below.)

If a conservator of the person is to be appointed for me, I nominate the following individual to serve as conservator of the person:

 Name: _____

 Address: _____

 Telephone:_____

8. CONTRIBUTION OF ANATOMICAL GIFT

(You may choose to make a gift of all or part of your body to a hospital, physician, or medical school for scientific, educational, therapeutic, or transplant purposes. Such a gift is allowed by California's Uniform Anatomical Gift Act. If you do not make such a gift, you may authorize your agent to do so, or a member of your family may make a gift unless you give them notice that you do not want a gift made. In the space below you may make a gift yourself or state that you do not want to make a gift. If you do not complete this section, your agent will have the authority to make a gift of all or a part of your body under the Uniform Anatomical Gift Act.)

If any of the statements below reflects your desires, sign on the line next to that statement. **You do not have to sign any of the statements.** If you do not sign any of the statements, your agent and your family will have the authority to make a gift of all or part of your body under the Uniform Anatomical Gift Act.

(_____)
(signature)   EXAMPLE

I have already signed a written agreement regarding anatomical gifts with the following individual or institution: _____

_____

(_____)
(signature)

Pursuant to the Uniform Anatomical Gift Act, I hereby give, effective upon my death

☐ Any needed organ or parts; or

☐ The parts or organs listed:

_____

_____

_____

for the following purpose (check one):

☐ Any legally authorized purpose

☐ Transplant/therapeutic purposes only and not for research

EXAMPLE

(_____)
(signature)

I do not want to make a gift under the Uniform Anatomical Gift Act, nor do I want my agent or family to do so.

9. AUTOPSY AND DISPOSITION OF MY REMAINS

I understand that my agent will be able to authorize an autopsy (an examination of my body after my death to determine the cause of my death) and to direct the disposition of my remains unless I limit that authority in this document. I also understand that my agent or any other person who directed the disposition of my remains must follow any instructions I have given in a written contract for funeral services, my will or by some other method.

(OPTIONAL: If you do not want your agent to be involved in these matters, you should state your desires concerning an autopsy and the person you would like to direct disposition of your remains. If any of the statements below reflect your desires, sign next to that statement. If none of these statements reflect your desires and you want to limit the authority of your agent to consent to an autopsy and/or to dispose of your remains, you should write your own statement in paragraph 4, above. Under some circumstances, the law may require that an autopsy be performed even if you have refused to authorize your agent to consent to one.)

Autopsy

(_____EXAMPLE_____)
(signature)

I hereby consent to an examination of my body after my death to determine the cause of my death.

(_____)
(signature)

My agent may not authorize an autopsy.

Disposition of Remains

(_____EXAMPLE_____)
(signature)

I prefer that my agent direct the disposition of my remains by the following method (check one) ☐ burial ☐ cremation

(_____)
(signature)

My agent may not direct the disposition of my remains and I would prefer that

_____
(name and address)

_____

(_____EXAMPLE_____)
(signature)

direct the disposition of my remains.

I have described the way I want my remains disposed of in (check one):
☐ A written contract for funeral services with

_____
(name of mortuary/cemetery)

☐ My will.

☐ Other: _____

10. PRIOR DESIGNATIONS REVOKED

I revoke any prior durable power of attorney for health care.

DATE AND SIGNATURE OF PRINCIPAL

(YOU MUST DATE AND SIGN THIS POWER OF ATTORNEY)

I sign my name to this Durable Power of Attorney for Health Care on _____ at

(Date)

_____ , _____

(City)   *(State)*

EXAMPLE

_____

(Signature of Principal)

(THIS POWER OF ATTORNEY WILL NOT BE VALID FOR MAKING HEALTH CARE DECISIONS UNLESS IT IS EITHER: (1) SIGNED BY TWO QUALIFIED ADULT WITNESSES WHO ARE PERSONALLY KNOWN TO YOU AND WHO ARE PRESENT WHEN YOU SIGN OR ACKNOWLEDGE YOUR SIGNATURE OR (2) ACKNOWLEDGED BEFORE A NOTARY PUBLIC IN CALIFORNIA.)

STATEMENT OF WITNESSES

(Unless you elect to have this document notarized, two qualified adult witnesses must complete this section. None of the following may be used as witnesses: (1) a person you designate as your agent or alternate agent, (2) a health care provider, (3) an employee of of a health care provider, (4) the operator of a community care facility or residential care facility for the elderly, (5) an employee of an operator of a community care facility or residential care facility for the elderly. At least one of the witnesses must make the additional declaration set out following the place where the witnesses sign.)

I declare under penalty of perjury under the laws of California that the person who signed or acknowledged this document is personally known to me to be the principal, that the principal signed or acknowledged this durable power of attorney in my presence, that the principal appears to be sound of mind and under no duress, fraud, or undue influence, that I am not the person appointed as attorney-in-fact by this document, and that I am not a health care provider, an employee of a health care provider, the operator of a community care facility or residential care facility for the elderly, nor an employee of an operator of a community care facility or residential care facility for the elderly.

Signature: _____   Residence Address: _____

Print Name: _____   _____

Date: _____   _____

Signature: _____   Residence Address: _____

Print Name: _____   _____

Date: _____   _____

(AT LEAST ONE OF THE ABOVE WITNESSES MUST ALSO SIGN THE FOLLOWING DECLARATION.)

I further declare under penalty of perjury under the laws of California that I am not related to the principal by blood, marriage, or adoption, and, to the best of my knowledge I am not entitled to any part of the estate of the principal upon the death of the principal under a will now existing or by operation of law.

Signature: _____ **EXAMPLE** _____

(Optional Second Signature): _____

COPIES

YOUR AGENT MAY NEED THIS DOCUMENT IMMEDIATELY IN CASE OF AN EMERGENCY THAT REQUIRES A DECISION CONCERNING YOUR HEALTH CARE. YOU SHOULD KEEP THE COMPLETED ORIGINAL DOCUMENT AND GIVE A COPY OF THE COMPLETED ORIGINAL TO YOUR AGENT AND ANY ALTERNATE AGENTS. YOU SHOULD ALSO GIVE A COPY TO YOUR DOCTOR, MEMBERS OF YOUR FAMILY, AND ANY OTHER PEOPLE WHO WOULD BE LIKELY TO NEED A COPY OF THIS FORM TO CARRY OUT YOUR WISHES. PHOTOCOPIES OF THIS DOCUMENT CAN BE RELIED UPON AS THOUGH THEY WERE ORIGINALS.

CERTIFICATE OF ACKNOWLEDGEMENT OF NOTARY PUBLIC

(You may use acknowledgement before a notary public instead of the statement of witnesses which appears on the preceding page.)

State of California ⟩

⟩ ss.

County of _____ ⟩

On this _____ day of _____ , in the year _____ ,

before me. _____ ,
(here insert name of notary public)

personally appeared _____
(here insert name of principal)

personally known to me (or proved to me on the basis of satisfactory evidence) to be the person whose name is subscribed to this instrument, and acknowledged that he or she executed it. I declare under penalty of perjury that the person whose name is subscribed to this instrument appears to be of sound mind and under no duress, fraud, or undue influence.

NOTARY SEAL

EXAMPLE

_____
(Signature of Notary Public)

SPECIAL REQUIREMENTS

(Special additional requirements must be satisfied for this document to be valid if (1) you are a patient in a skilled nursing facility or (2) you are a conservatee under the Lanterman-Petris-Short Act and you are appointing your conservator as your agent to make health care decisions for you. If you are not sure whether you are in a skilled nursing facility, which is a special type of nursing home, ask the facility staff. If you are not sure whether the person you want to choose as your health care agent is your conservator under the Lanterman-Petris-Short Act, ask that person.)

1. If you are in a skilled nursing facility (as defined in Health and Safety Code Section 1250(c)) at least one of the witnesses must be a patient advocate or ombudsman. The patient advocate or ombudsman must sign the witness statement and must also sign the following declaration:

I further declare under penalty of perjury under the laws of California that I am a patient advocate or ombudsman as designated by the State Department of Aging and am serving as a witness as required by subdivision (f) of Civil Code Section 2432.

Signature: _____ Address: _____

Print Name: _____ _____

Date: _____ _____

If you are a conservatee under the Lanterman-Petris-Short Act (of Division 5 of the Welfare and Institutions Code) and you wish to designate your conservator as your agent to make health care decisions, you must be represented by legal counsel. Your lawyer must also sign the following statement:

I am a lawyer authorized to practice law in the state where this power of attorney was executed, and the principal was my client at the time this power of attorney was executed. I have advised my client concerning his or her rights in connection with this power of attorney and the applicable law and the consequences of signing or not signing this power of attorney, and my client, after being so advised, has executed this power of attorney.

Signature: _____ Address: _____

Print Name: _____ _____

Date: _____ _____

12

Getting the Most Out
of Medicines

Having HIV/AIDS usually means taking one or more medications. Thus a very important self-management task is to understand your medications and to use them appropriately. This chapter will help you do just that.

A Few General Words
About Medications

Almost nothing receives as much advertising as medications. If we read a magazine, listen to the radio, or watch TV, we are bombarded with a constant stream of ads, all aimed to convince us that if we just use this pill or potion, our symptoms will be cured. "Recommended by 90 percent of the doctors asked." "Take an aspirin for your headache." Almost as a backlash to this advertising, we have been taught to avoid excess medications. We have all heard about or experienced some of the ill effects of medications. "Just say no to drugs." "Drugs can kill." It is all very confusing.

Your body is its own healer, and if it is given time to work this healing, many common symptoms and disorders will improve. The prescriptions filled by the body's internal pharmacy are frequently the safest and most effective treatment. So patience, careful self-observation, and self-monitoring are excellent therapeutic choices.

It is also true that medications are a very important part of managing HIV/AIDS. So far, medications can not cure the disease, but they generally have one or more of the following purposes:

- They *help symptoms* through their chemical actions. For example, pain medications decrease activity in nerve cells, which can decrease pain sensations. Nausea medications decrease stomach hyperactivity, quieting stomach upset.

- Other medications help to *prevent further problems*. For example, people with high risk for *Pneumocystis* pneumonia take medicines to prevent the pneumonia from starting.

- A third type of medication helps to *improve the disease or slow the disease process*. For example, anti-HIV drugs like AZT (Zidovudine; Retrovir) or ddI (didanosine; Videx) can slow the effects of HIV on the immune system.

- Finally, there are medications to *replace substances that the body is no longer producing adequately*. Blood transfusions are a "medication" of this type.

In all cases, the purpose of medication is to lessen the consequences of disease or to slow its course. However, as you can see, many of the drugs we use will not have an obvious positive effect that you can detect when you take them. Sometimes the drug will keep a condition stable when without the drug it would have worsened. Sometimes the drug may only slow down a deterioration that would have been more rapid without the drug. It can be easy to think that the drug isn't doing anything. But except for drugs that are taken *just* for symptoms, it's hard to judge just by how you feel whether medications are working or not. That's why it's important to talk openly with your doctor about your medications and discuss any changes you might want to make.

Besides being helpful, all medications have undesirable side effects. Some are predictable and minor, and some are unexpected and life threatening. From 5 to 10 percent of all hospital admissions are due to drug reactions. But in spite of this, there's no reason to be frightened of medications. By knowing what medications you're using and by knowing what (and what not) to expect, you can maximize your benefit and reduce the chance of serious side effects.

What Is a Side Effect?

A side effect is any effect other than the one you want. Usually, it is an undesirable effect. Examples of undesirable side effects are stomach problems, constipation, diarrhea, sleepiness, or dizziness. You should know the common side effects of the medications you take. Sometimes people say they can't or won't take a drug because of possible side effects. This is a reasonable response. However, before making a decision to stop a drug or refusing to take it, you should ask yourself and your doctor the following questions.

Are the benefits from this medication more important than the side effects?

The drugs used to treat cancer (chemotherapy) are a good example of medications whose benefits you may want to weigh against their undesirable side effects. Although these drugs have side effects, many people still choose the drugs because of their life-saving qualities. To take or not to take a drug is your decision. However, you should always ask yourself, "Will I be better off with the drug despite its side effects?"

Are there some ways of avoiding the side effects or making them less severe?

Many times the way you take the drug—for example, with or without food—can make a difference. Ask your doctor or pharmacist for advice on this question.

Are there other medications with the same benefits but fewer side effects?

Often several drugs do the same thing but react differently in different people. Unfortunately, no one knows how a drug will react in you until you have taken it. Therefore your doctor may have to try several medications before hitting on the one that is best for you. For this reason, when getting a new medication, it is always best to ask for a prescription that will last only a week or two, with a refill for a month. In this way, if the drug does not work out, you will not have had to pay for a large amount of medication that you do not use.

Monitoring Medications

It is common for people with HIV to be taking multiple medications: anti-HIV medications, anti-inflammatory drugs for pain or fever, a pill for depression, an antibiotic to prevent *Pneumocystis*, antacids for heartburn, a tranquilizer for anxiety, plus a handful of over-the-counter (OTC) remedies. *Remember, the more medications you are taking, the greater the risk of adverse reactions.* Fortunately, you can often reduce the number of medications and the associated risks if you have forged an effective partnership with your doctor.

Such a relationship requires your participation in determining the need for the medication, selecting the medication, properly using the medication, and reporting back to your doctor the effect of the medication.

An individual's response to a particular medication varies depending upon age, metabolism, activity level, and the waxing and waning of symptoms characteristic of most HIV diseases. Many medications are prescribed on an as-needed ("PRN") basis, so you need to know when to begin and end treatment and how much medication to take. You need to work out a plan with your doctor to suit your individual needs.

For most medications, *your doctor depends on you* to report what effect, if any, the drug has on your symptoms and what side effects you may be experiencing. On the basis of that critical information, your doctor may continue, increase, discontinue, or otherwise change your medications. A good doctor/patient partnership requires a continuing flow of information. There are important things you need to let your doctor know and critical information you need to receive in return.

Unfortunately, this vital interchange is too often short-changed. Studies indicate that fewer than 5 percent of patients receiving new prescriptions asked any questions of their physicians or pharmacists. Doctors tend to interpret patient silence as understanding and satisfaction with the information received. Mishaps often occur because patients either do not receive adequate information about medications and don't understand how to take them or fail to follow instructions given to them. Safe, effective drug use depends on your understanding of the proper use, the risks, and the necessary precautions associated with each medication you take. *You must ask questions.*

Some people are reluctant to ask their doctor questions because they are afraid of appearing ignorant or of challenging the doctor's authority. But asking questions is a necessary part of a healthy doctor/patient relationship.

The goal of treatment is to maximize the benefits and minimize the risks. Whether the medications you take are helpful or harmful often depends on how much you know about your medications and how well you communicate with your doctor.

What You Need to Tell Your Doctor

Even if your doctor doesn't ask, there is certain vital information you should mention to him or her.

Are you taking any medications?

Report to your physician and dentist *all* the prescription and nonprescription medications you are taking, including experimental medicines, herbs, birth control pills, vitamins, aspirin, antacids, and laxatives. This information is especially important if you are seeing more than one physician because each one may not know what the others have prescribed. Knowing all the medications you are taking is essential for correct diagnosis and treatment. For example, symptoms such as nausea, diarrhea, sleeplessness, drowsiness, dizziness, memory loss, impotence, or fatigue may be due to a drug side effect rather than a disease. It is critical for your doctor to know what medications you are taking to help avoid problems from drug interactions. Carry an up-to-date list with you, or at least know the names and dosages of all the medications you are taking. Saying that you are taking "the little green pills" usually doesn't help identify the medication. Everyone should get into the habit of doing a "brown bag" medicine check at least once every six months. The idea is simple: put all the medicines you're taking into a bag and bring them in with you when you see your doctor. Review *all* the medicines with your doctor and make sure you know which to continue and which to stop or discard. Don't forget the over-the-counter and the "as needed" medications!

Have you had allergic or unusual reactions to any medications?

Describe any symptoms or unusual reactions you have had to any medications taken in the past. Be specific: which medication and exactly what type of reaction. A rash, fever, or wheezing that develops after taking a medication is often a true allergic reaction. If any of these develop, call your doctor at once. Nausea, ringing in the ears, lightheadedness, and agitation are likely to be side effects rather than true drug allergies.

*Do you have any major chronic diseases or medical conditions
other than HIV?*

Many diseases can interfere with the action of a drug or increase the risk of using certain medications. Diseases involving the kidneys or liver are especially important to mention since these diseases can slow the metabolism of many drugs and increase toxic effects. Your doctor may also avoid certain medications if you now have or in the past have had such diseases as hypertension, peptic ulcer disease, asthma, heart disease, diabetes, or prostate problems. Also be sure to let your doctor know if you are possibly pregnant or are breast-feeding, since many drugs cannot be safely used in those situations.

What medications were tried in the past to treat your disease?

If you have a chronic symptom or symptoms, it is a good idea to keep your own written record of what medications were tried in the past to manage the condition and what the effects were. Knowing your past responses to various medications will help guide the doctor's recommendation of any new medications. However, just because a medication did not work successfully in the past does not necessarily mean that it can't be tried again. Diseases change and may become more responsive to treatment.

What You Need
to Ask Your Doctor

Do I really need this medication?

Some physicians decide to prescribe medications not because they are really necessary, but because they think patients want and expect drugs. Physicians often feel pressure to do something for the patient, so they reach for the prescription pad. Don't pressure your physician for medications. If your doctor doesn't prescribe a medication, consider that good news rather than a sign of rejection or disinterest. Ask about nondrug alternatives. Many conditions can be treated in a variety of ways, and your physician can explain alternative choices. In some cases, lifestyle changes such as exercise, diet, and stress management should be considered before making a choice. When any treatment is recommended, also ask what the likely consequences are if you postpone treatment. Sometimes the best medicine is none at all.

What is the name of the medication?

If a medication is prescribed, it is important that you know its name. Write down both the brand name and the generic (chemical) name. If the medication you get from the pharmacy doesn't have the same name as the one your doctor prescribed, ask the pharmacist to explain the difference.

What is the medication supposed to do?

Your doctor should tell you why the medication is being prescribed and how it might be expected to help you. Is the medication intended to prolong your life, completely or partially relieve your symptoms, or improve your ability to function? For example, if you are given an anti-HIV drug like AZT (Retrovir), the purpose is primarily to prevent or slow down deterioration of your immune system. It probably won't stop your HIV-related symptoms, and it may give you side effects. On the other hand, if you are given a skin cream, the purpose is to help ease your skin condition. You should also know how soon you should expect results from the medication. Drugs that treat infections or inflammation may take several days to a week to show improvement, whereas antidepressant medications typically take several weeks to begin working.

How and when do I take the medication, and for how long?

Understanding how much of the medication to take and how often to take it is critical to the safe, effective use of medications. Does "every 6 hours" mean "every 6 hours while awake?" Should the medication be taken before meals, with meals, or between meals? What should you do if you accidentally miss a dose? Should you skip it, take a double dose next time, or take it as soon as you remember? Should you continue taking the medication until the symptoms subside or until the medication is finished?

The answers to such questions are very important. For example, if you are taking an antibiotic for a lung infection, you may feel better within a few days, but you should still take the medication as prescribed to completely eliminate the infection. Otherwise, the infection may come back, perhaps in a stronger, drug-resistant form. Didanosine (ddI, Videx) has to be taken two pills at a time and chewed or crushed in order to be effective. If you are using an inhaled medication for treatment of breathing problems, the way you use the inhaler critically determines how much of the medication actually gets into your lungs. Taking medication properly is vital. Yet when patients are surveyed, nearly 40 percent report that they were not told by their physicians how to take the medication or how much to take. If you are not sure about your prescription, call your doctor. Such calls are never considered a bother.

What foods, drinks, other medications, or activities should I avoid while taking this medication?

The presence of food in the stomach may help protect the stomach from some medications, whereas it may render other drugs ineffective. For example, milk products or antacids can decrease the absorption of some antibiotics (like Nizoral) but may increase the absorption of others. Some medications may make you more sensitive to the sun, putting you at increased risk for sunburn. Ask whether the medication prescribed will interfere with driving safely. Other drugs you may be taking, even over-the-counter drugs and alcohol, can either amplify or inhibit the effects of the prescribed medication. Taking aspirin if you have decreased platelet function can result in enhanced blood-thinning and possible bleeding. The more medications you are taking, the greater the chance of undesirable drug interactions. So ask about possible drug-and-drug and drug-food interactions.

*What are the most common side effects, and what should
I do if they occur?*

All medications have side effects. You need to know what symptoms to be
on the lookout for and what action to take if they develop. Should you seek
immediate medical care, discontinue the medication, or call your doctor?
Although your doctor cannot be expected to tell you every possible adverse
reaction, the more common and important ones should be discussed.
Unfortunately, a recent survey showed that 70 percent of patients starting a
new medication did not recall being told by their physicians or pharmacists
about precautions and possible side effects. So it may be up to you to ask.

Are there any tests necessary to monitor the use of this medication?

Some medications are monitored by the improvement or worsening of
symptoms. However, many medications used to treat people with HIV can
disrupt body chemistry before any telltale symptoms develop. Sometimes
these adverse reactions can be detected by laboratory tests such as blood
counts or liver function tests. In addition, the levels of some medications in
the blood need to be measured periodically to make sure you are getting the
right amounts. Ask your doctor if the medication being prescribed has any of
these special requirements.

Can a generic medication that is less expensive be prescribed?

Every drug has at least two names, a generic name and a brand name. The
generic name is the nonproprietary, or chemical, name of the drug. The
brand name is the manufacturer's unique name for the drug. When a drug
company develops a new drug in the United States, it is granted exclusive
rights to produce that drug for seventeen years. After this seventeen-year
period has expired, other companies may market chemical equivalents of that
drug. These generic medications are generally considered as safe and effective
as the original brand-name drug but often cost half as much. Because many
AIDS drugs are quite new, often no generic equivalent is available. Even so, if
cost is a concern, ask your doctor if there is a lower-cost, but equally effective,
medication. Sometimes you can save money by purchasing your medications
through the mail. Many health maintenance organizations (HMOs) and mail-
order pharmacies offer prescription services.

Is there any written information about the medication?

Realistically, your doctor may not have time to answer all of your questions in great detail. Even if your physician carefully answers the questions, it
is difficult for anyone to remember all this information. Fortunately, there are

many other valuable sources of information you can turn to: pharmacists, nurses, package inserts, pamphlets, and books. Several particularly useful publications to consult are listed under "Suggested Reading" at the end of this chapter.

A Special Word About Pharmacists

Pharmacists are an underutilized resource. They have gone to school for many years to learn about medications, how they act in your body, and how they interact with each other. Your pharmacist is an expert on medications. You can often call him or her on the phone. In addition, many hospitals, medical schools, and schools of pharmacy have medication information services where you can call and ask questions. As a self-manager, don't forget pharmacists. They are important and helpful consultants.

Remembering to Take Your Medicine

No matter what medication is prescribed, it won't do you any good if you don't take it. Nearly half of all medicines are not taken regularly as prescribed. The reasons are many: forgetfulness, lack of clear instructions, complicated dosing schedules, bothersome side effects, cost of the medications, and so on. Whatever the reason, if you are having trouble taking your medications as prescribed, discuss the problem with your doctor. Often simple adjustments can make it easier. For example, if you are taking five different medications, perhaps some can be eliminated. If you are taking one medication three times a day and another four times a day, your doctor may be able to simplify the regimen, perhaps even prescribing medications that you only need to take once or twice a day. If cost is a significant barrier, be frank with your doctor. Often another effective, but less expensive, medication can be substituted. Understanding more about your medications, including how they can help you, may also help motivate you to take them regularly.

If forgetting to take your medications is a major problem, the following suggestions may help:

- *Place the medication or a reminder next to your toothbrush*, on the meal table, in your lunch box, or in some other place where you're likely to "stumble over" it. (But be careful where you put the medication if children are around.) Or you might put a reminder note on the bathroom mirror, the refrigerator door, the coffeemaker, the television, or some other conspicuous place. If you link taking the medication with some well-established habit like mealtimes or watching your favorite TV program, you'll be more likely to remember.

- *Make a medication chart* containing each medication you are taking and when you take it; or check off each medication on a calendar as you take it. You might also *buy a medication organizer* at the drugstore. This container separates pills according to the time of day they should be taken. You can fill the organizer once a week so all of your pills are ready to take at the proper time. A quick glance at the organizer lets you know if you have missed any doses and prevents double dosing.

- *Get a watch that can be set to beep at pill-taking time.* There are also high-tech medication containers available that beep at a preprogrammed time to remind you to take your medication.

- *Ask other family or household members to help remind you* to take your medications.

- *Don't let yourself run out* of your medicines. When you get a new prescription, mark on your calendar the date a week before your medications will run out. This will serve as a reminder to get your next refill. Don't wait until the last pill.

- If you plan to travel, *put a note on your luggage reminding you* to pack your pills. Also, *take along an extra prescription* in your carry-on luggage in case you lose your pills or your luggage.

Self-Medication

In addition to medications prescribed by your doctor, you, like most people, probably take nonprescription or over-the-counter (OTC) medications. In fact, within every 2-week period nearly 70 percent of people will self-medicate with one or more drugs. Many over-the-counter drugs are highly effective and may even be recommended by your doctor. But if you self-medicate, you should know what you are taking, why you are taking it, how it works, and how to use medications wisely.

More than 200,000 nonprescription drug products, representing about 500 active ingredients, are offered for sale to the American public, which spends an estimated $8 billion per year on such products. Nearly 75 percent of the public receives its education on over-the-counter drugs solely from

TV, radio, newspaper, and magazine advertising. Unfortunately, many of the claims for such drugs are either not true or subtly misleading.

You need to be aware of the barrage of drug advertising aimed at you. The implicit message of such advertising is that for every symptom, every ache and pain, every problem, there is a product solution. Although many of the OTC products are effective, many are simply a waste of your money and a diversion of your attention from better ways of managing your illness.

If you self-medicate, the following suggestions will help you do so safely:

- *Always read drug labels and follow directions carefully.* The label must by law include names and quantities of the active ingredients, precautions, and adequate directions for safe use. Careful reading of the label, including review of the individual ingredients, may help prevent you from ingesting medications that have caused problems for you in the past. If you don't understand the information on the label, ask a pharmacist or doctor before buying it.

- *Do not exceed the recommended dosage or length of treatment* unless you discuss it with your doctor.

- *Use caution if you are taking other medications.* Over-the-counter and prescription drugs can interact, either canceling or exaggerating the effects of the medications. If you have questions about drug interactions, ask your doctor or pharmacist before mixing medicines.

- Try to *select medications with single active ingredients* rather than the combination ("all-in-one") products. In using a product with multiple ingredients, you are likely to be getting drugs for symptoms you don't even have, so why risk the side effects of medications you don't need? Single-ingredient products also allow you to adjust the dosage of each medication separately for optimal symptom relief with minimal side effects.

- When choosing medications, *learn the ingredient names* and try to *buy generic products.* Generics contain the same active ingredient as the brand-name product, usually at a lower cost.

- *Never take or give a drug from an unlabeled container* or a container whose label you cannot read. Keep your medications in their original, labeled containers or transfer them to a labeled medication organizer or pill dispenser. Do not make the mistake of mixing different medications in the same bottle.

- *Do not take medications left over* from a previous illness or that were prescribed for someone else, even if you have similar symptoms. Always check out medications with your doctor.

- Pills can sometimes get stuck in your esophagus (the "feeding tube" between your throat and your stomach). To help prevent this, be sure to *drink at least a half glass of liquid* with your pills and remain standing or sitting upright for a few minutes after swallowing.

- If you are pregnant or nursing, have liver or kidney trouble, or are taking other medications, *consult your doctor* before self-medicating.

- *Store your medications in a safe place* away from the reach of children. Poisoning with medications is a common and preventable problem. The bathroom medicine chest is not automatically a particularly secure or dry place to store medications. Consider a lockable tool chest or fishing box.

- Many medications have an expiration date of 2 to 3 years. *Dispose of all expired medications.*

Medications can help or harm. What often makes the difference is the care you exercise and the partnership you develop with your doctor.

Nonapproved Therapies

Although treatment for HIV/AIDS has improved greatly during the last ten years, none of the therapies now approved by the Food and Drug Administration (FDA) is a cure. For this reason, there is much interest in identifying and developing new and innovative treatments for HIV/AIDS. Different treatments are being suggested all the time. It often seems that every week something gets publicity as the next big treatment. Some nonapproved therapies are *experimental therapies*—drugs still in development or not yet approved for human use. Others are *"alternative" therapies*—diets, herbs, vitamins, or other holistic approaches.

How should anyone decide about whether to use a treatment that is not officially FDA-approved? How can you make a decision about which of the various treatments to use? There is no absolute answer, but you need to get the best and most reliable information you can.

Fortunately, there are several good ways to get information about experimental and alternative therapies. Your doctors and nurses are always a good place to start. Even if they aren't experts on the specific remedy you're interested in, they can point you toward sources where you'll be able to learn more. Project Inform is a national organization devoted specifically to educating people about different HIV/AIDS treatments. They have a 24-hour telephone hotline for questions and have published an excellent book (*The HIV Drug Book*) featuring information on all kinds of therapies. If you have access to a computer, the Internet has volumes of information about therapies. The World Wide Web has so many HIV/AIDS-related resources that they're difficult to keep up with.

But after you've gathered all the information you can find, how should you finally decide? Talk to your doctor or nurse practitioner. Talk to your local AIDS organization. Talk to other people who know about the treatment you're considering. But keep in mind that it may not be valid to put too much weight on the "miracle cure" that *one* person got from a certain drug. Often, people talk more about successes than failures. From the enthusiasts, you won't hear about the *other* people, who had bad experiences with the same drug. Finally, try to weigh the risks and benefits of using the alternative treatment. Do what seems to make sense for you.

Experimental Therapies

Many people are interested in participating in official experimental studies of new treatments for HIV/AIDS. Experimental therapies are drugs that are not yet proven to work, but which are being scientifically studied for their effects. If you are part of an experimental study, you may be one of the first people to get a new and improved treatment. But you may also get no benefit at all over standard therapies. The study organizers are required to fully inform you about the pluses and minuses of participating. Get the best information you can by discussing the therapy you are considering with your doctor, Project Inform, and friends.

Consider the following advantages and drawbacks, which apply to all experimental scientific studies:

Advantages

- The treatment will be medically and scientifically supervised.
- Since a study is being done, the treatment already has some scientific evidence to support it.
- You may help to develop new, better treatments that will help others.

Drawbacks

- Many of the treatments being studied have side effects; some may do more harm than good.

- In some studies, you may receive a placebo (a medicine with no physical effect).
- So you won't confuse the results, you may be asked not to use certain other treatments while you are in the study.
- Being in a study can take time and effort.

After weighing the information, make the best decision you can. And as always, cooperate and get help from your doctor in this process.

"Alternative" Therapies

Many "alternative" (or complementary) treatments are being suggested all the time for use outside of any experimental study. These treatments are often herbal or holistic and are usually (though not always) fairly safe.

Which of these alternative treatments are effective? Unfortunately, there are no easy answers. On the one hand, many unofficial but highly publicized treatments over the years have turned out to be ineffective, and a few have even been harmful. On the other hand, some alternative treatments may well turn out to be helpful. Several accepted treatments (like ddI and ddC) were first available unofficially through buyers' clubs. In certain situations, and for certain people, it may be reasonable to consider using an alternative treatment. Here are some practical tips for evaluating nonapproved, alternative treatments:*

- *Is someone trying to sell you something?* Watch out for the words *amazing* or *miraculous.* No responsible scientist would use these words.
- *Does the product contain secret ingredients?* If the ingredients are secret, then there's no way for anyone to tell what the product is or what it does.
- *Do promoters use pseudoscience to help sell the product?* Watch out for scientific-sounding lingo that is difficult to understand.
- *Is the product sold only through the mail?* This can be a sign of trouble.
- *Is there a possibility that this treatment could be harmful?*
- *Is this treatment expensive?* Can you afford it?

---

*Adapted from John S. James, in *AIDS Treatment News,* and Jill A. Jarvie, in *Positive Nutrition.*

Suggested Reading

About Your Medicines. United States Pharmacopeial Convention, 1989.

AIDS Treatment News. ATN, P.O. Box 411256, San Francisco, CA 94141. (A semi-monthly newsletter reporting on HIV/AIDS treatments.) Published by John S. James.

The American Medical Association Guide to Prescription and Over-the-Counter Drugs. Edited by Charles Clayman. New York: Random House, 1988.

Long, James W. *The Essential Guide to Prescription Drugs.* New York: Harper & Row, 1989.

Petrow, Steven (ed). *The HIV Drug Book.* New York: Pocket Books, 1995. (The only reference available that lists and describes all the drugs used by people with HIV, their effects, and their interactions.)

Resources

Finding Out about Alternative Therapies

Project Inform Drug Information Hotline
1-800-822-7422

13

Understanding AIDS and the Immune System

What exactly is AIDS? AIDS is a disease of the immune system caused by a virus, the human immunodeficiency virus, or HIV. People who become infected with HIV develop damage to their immune system gradually over a period of years. When the immune damage is minimal, a person with HIV doesn't notice anything at all. If the immune damage gets worse, the person may notice swollen lymph nodes or get certain mild infections of the skin or mouth. If the immune damage gets quite severe, people with HIV lose the ability to fight off serious infections and cancers that otherwise wouldn't cause much trouble. If one or more of these serious infections or cancers develops, the person is said to have AIDS: Acquired Immune Deficiency Syndrome.

In the next several pages, we will cover some detailed information: how HIV is (and isn't) transmitted, what HIV does to the immune system, what illnesses HIV can cause, and what tests and treatments are commonly used in caring for HIV/AIDS. Some readers may find this information frightening, but it's impossible to be a self-manager without knowledge of the basics. Knowing medical details about HIV/AIDS should not lead you to lose track of three vital overall facts:

- HIV/AIDS is treatable. People in treatment are living longer and better now than ever in the past.

- Treatments for HIV/AIDS are improving all the time. People starting treatment now have more and better therapy options than ever before.

- Everyone with HIV/AIDS has a unique experience. People can give you probabilities, but no one can say what will happen to you. For example, it's a mistake to assume that because your friend got *Pneumocystis* (PCP) and dementia that you will automatically get those same diseases.

182

How Do People Catch AIDS?

Since AIDS is really the advanced form of infection with HIV, the real question is, How do people catch HIV infection? Since HIV only infects humans, the only way to transmit HIV is for the virus to travel from inside one person who is already infected into the blood stream of another person. Now remember, some viruses, such as influenza (flu), concentrate in the lungs, so *coughing* spreads them around. Other viruses, such as chicken pox, concentrate in the skin, so *touching* an infected person leads to spread of the disease. HIV is different; it concentrates primarily in the blood and semen, and there aren't many ways to transfer blood and semen from one person to another.

Because HIV concentrates primarily in the blood and semen, nearly all the known cases of HIV infection have been transmitted in one of the following ways:

- sexual contact
- sharing of contaminated intravenous (IV) needles
- passage of the virus from mother to unborn child
- transfusions of blood or blood products

Sexual Contact

For an HIV-positive person to have unprotected sex is risky, but exactly how risky depends on exactly what you do during sex. Unprotected anal intercourse appears to be the most effective way to transmit HIV sexually. When a person with HIV puts his bare penis into another person's anus, the receiving person, whether a man or a woman, is at high risk for catching HIV. Unprotected vaginal intercourse is also risky, though probably a bit less risky than unprotected anal intercourse, since less cracking and bleeding of the skin occurs.

There are two reasons why it is vital to practice safe sex if you are HIV positive:

- *To protect others.* Obviously, you would not want to expose someone else to a serious illness.
- *To protect yourself.* Even if you are already HIV positive, you can be reinfected with new, possibly more dangerous strains of HIV. Your chances of disease progression may be less if you can avoid reinfection. People with HIV are also at increased risk to get other important sexually transmitted diseases—such as syphilis, gonorrhea, and hepatitis—through unsafe sex.

Needles and Syringes

HIV-infected people who use a needle and syringe (the plastic container attached to the needle) for injecting drugs leave a small amount of blood in the needle or syringe after they're done. If the needle or syringe is then used by someone else without being sterilized, the first person's blood can be injected into the next person, causing transfer of the infection.

Mother to Child

The *placenta* is an organ inside a pregnant woman that allows food and oxygen from the mother to go to the baby inside her. If an HIV-positive woman is pregnant, the HIV in her blood can cross the barrier of the placenta to get into her baby's blood while the child is still in the womb. This kind of HIV transmission seems to happen in about one-third of babies born to HIV-positive mothers. When it does happen, the baby will be born infected with HIV.

Blood Transfusion

Since HIV is concentrated in blood, blood transfusion was an important source of transmission until the blood test for HIV became available in 1985. Before 1985, blood banks couldn't tell which of the blood units they received had HIV and therefore were dangerous to give to others. Now the risk of getting HIV from a blood transfusion is low, but not zero. Although the blood test for HIV is extremely good, it's not perfect. Also, people *newly* infected with HIV won't develop signs of HIV in the blood for about 3–6 months, so HIV-infected blood could be collected during this period and not be detected by the tests. But again, most people with HIV from blood transfusions were exposed before 1985. The chances of transmitting HIV through a blood transfusion now are extremely remote.

Possible Other Ways

Everyone agrees about how risky it is to have unprotected sex or share dirty hypodermic needles between an HIV-positive and an HIV-negative person. But certain other activities are harder to be sure about. Kissing deeply with exchange of saliva is a good example. No cases of HIV infection due to kissing have ever been proven. Saliva contains extremely low concentrations of HIV, so infection from saliva seems unlikely. But because of sores, bleeding gums, and bites, blood in the mouth is common and not always easy to see. In theory, this blood could transmit HIV. In practice, however, no confirmed cases have been identified.

Ways of Catching HIV from an HIV-Positive Person		
Definitely Risky	*Low Risk*	*Not Risky*
Unprotected anal sex	Mouth-to-genitals sex	Shaking hands
Unprotected vaginal sex	Kissing with saliva exchange	Sharing bathroom
Sharing unclean needles	Sharing razor or toothbrush	Touching doorknobs
Mouth-to-anus sex		Casual social contact
		Contact with sweat
		Insects

What Does HIV Infection Do?

People who are infected with HIV experience a slow deterioration of their immune system. The immune system is vital to proper functioning of the human body, and that's why people with HIV infection can have so much trouble. The human immune system has many different components: there are infection-fighting white blood cells; there are messenger chemicals that signal parts of the system to turn on and off depending on what invader is causing problems; there are natural human toxins ("killer" chemicals) that can destroy invading organisms; and there are proteins that can "tag" invaders, making them more easily attacked by the rest of the immune system. All of the parts of the immune system are important, but HIV particularly attacks one part of the immune system, a type of white blood cell called *T cells* (also called *T helper*, *T4*, or *CD4 cells*). People with HIV/AIDS have problems with certain specific types of infections and cancer types—the infections and cancer types ordinarily controlled by good T cell function.

HIV can also infect brain cells, cells inside the bones (the bone marrow), and cells in the lining of the intestines. Because of the effect on brain cells, some people develop confusion and memory problems if their condition is quite advanced. Since blood cells are made in the bone marrow, the effect of HIV on the bone marrow can lead to decreased blood counts (anemia). Chronic problems with diarrhea may come from the effect of HIV on the intestines.

The average time from infection with HIV to developing full-blown AIDS is eleven years. This is an estimated average time for everyone with HIV, so some people will develop AIDS sooner and some later. No one can predict what will happen to any one individual.

Basically, HIV infection can be divided into four stages:

1. the healthy carrier state
2. the enlarged lymph node stage (lymphadenopathy syndrome)
3. AIDS-related complex (ARC)
4. AIDS

In the healthy carrier state, people have no symptoms of any kind and really do not feel different from normal. Unfortunately, even at this stage, HIV-positive people can transmit the virus to others. People who develop the lymphadenopathy syndrome have swollen lymph nodes that persist for many months without any other signs of infection. At this stage, some people also have mild symptoms of tiredness or unexplained fevers. AIDS-related complex (ARC) indicates more advanced HIV infection—people with ARC generally feel as if they have a chronic illness that limits life to some degree. ARC-related symptoms and conditions include oral thrush (a white, cottage cheese-like mouth infection), skin infections, and blood test abnormalities, among others. AIDS is the most advanced of the four stages of HIV infection; people with AIDS have a lot of damage to their T cells and immune system. If the damage gets severe enough, HIV-positive people may develop certain infections or cancers, and if they do, they are said to have progressed to AIDS.

Illnesses Associated with AIDS and ARC

Most of the severe problems that come from having HIV are caused by the infections and cancers that people can get when the immune system gets weak. The most common illnesses are discussed below.

Pneumocystis carinii Pneumonia (PCP)

Pneumonia (lung infection) caused by the parasite *Pneumocystis carinii* is the most common AIDS-related illness in the United States. Over half of all AIDS patients get pneumocystis and over 80 percent of HIV-infected people who *don't* take a preventive medicine can expect to get the disease. *Pneumocystis* initially caused up to 50 percent of the AIDS deaths in this country, but now better curative and preventive medications are available. Preventive therapy involves treating people at high risk for getting PCP with low doses of PCP drugs so that they never get the disease. This approach has saved many people.

Kaposi's Sarcoma (KS)

Kaposi's sarcoma is a type of slow-growing skin cancer that initially appears as a purple, brown, or pink bump on the skin. It may be very limited and not cause much trouble, but sometimes it can spread widely on the skin and even spread to the internal organs. KS is seen primarily in gay men—it's rare in heterosexuals, even in IV drug users. When it's mild, KS may not need any treatment. But in severe cases, anticancer drugs (chemotherapy) may be needed.

Toxoplasmosis of the Brain

Toxoplasmosis is caused by a parasite (*Toxoplasma gondii*) found in undercooked meat and is a common infection of humans as well as many animals. Toxoplasma is also often found in cat litter boxes, in dirt, and in other places where animals leave their wastes. Because of this, people with HIV/AIDS need to be careful about wearing gloves when changing cat litter or working in the garden. Usually "toxo" causes very few problems—most peoples' immune system controls the infection without any trouble. But in people with AIDS, the infection tends to go to the brain and cause strength, speech, seizure, or walking problems. Sometimes it can go to the internal organs as

AIDS- and ARC-Associated Illnesses

ARC	*AIDS*
Oral candida (thrush)	*Pneumocystis carinii* pneumonia
Oral hairy leukoplakia	Kaposi's sarcoma
Peripheral neuropathy	Toxoplasmosis of the brain
Chronic sinusitis	Cryptococcus meningitis
Idiopathic thrombocytopenic purpura	Cytomegalovirus (CMV) retinitis
Herpes zoster (shingles)	*Mycobacterium* infection (MAI or MAC)
Chronic folliculitis	Tuberculosis
Chronic dermatitis	Lymphoma
Chronic unexplained fever	Cryptosporidium diarrhea
Chronic unexplained diarrhea	Candida of the esophagus
	AIDS-related dementia
	AIDS wasting syndrome

well. If it's caught early enough, Toxoplasmosis can be controlled by taking oral medicines.

Mycobacterium avium Complex (MAC) or *Mycobacterium avium intracellulare* (MAI)

Mycobacterium avium is a bacterium that can spread widely through the blood and internal organs of people with AIDS. It generally isn't a danger until the T cell count is quite low, less than 100. By itself, MAC usually is not fatal, but it does weaken people a great deal. Symptoms, sometimes severe, include fevers, weight loss, sweats, swollen lymph nodes, diarrhea, and/or abdominal pains. Treating MAC requires taking two or three different types of antibiotics for long periods, perhaps indefinitely.

Candida

Candida is a fungus that is commonly found in the mouth, skin, gastrointestinal tract, and vagina. Candida of the mouth (thrush) and vagina is most common. It looks like white spots or patches that can be easily scraped off with a stick. When candida is in the esophagus (the swallowing tube to the stomach), it can be painful to swallow. For some people, finding thrush is the first sign of problems with the immune system. Fortunately, candida is usually easy to treat.

Cytomegalovirus (CMV)

Cytomegalovirus (CMV) is a very common virus that most people have been exposed to long before they are exposed to HIV. Only when the immune system is weakened does CMV start to cause problems in the eyes, intestinal tract, and sometimes other internal organs. CMV can damage the backs of the eyes (CMV retinitis), causing partial loss of vision and even blindness when it's very severe. In the intestinal tract (CMV colitis or enteritis), CMV causes pain, ulcers, bleeding, and diarrhea. Like MAC, CMV is mostly seen when the T cell count has dropped below 100. Medications can slow, and sometimes even stop the problems caused by CMV, but most of the medications require an IV (intravenous line) in your arm or chest.

Cryptococcosis

In cryptococcosis, a fungus (*Cryptococcus neoformans*) can cause meningitis, an infection of the lining of the brain. When it does, people often get fevers and headaches that are much more severe than usual, and sometimes they may have decreased consciousness. Much more rarely, *Cryptococcus* can also cause pneumonia and skin infections. The fungus may be transmitted by bird droppings, but it is widespread among humans and other mammals. The infection is treated with intravenous (IV) medication when it's severe, but in its mild form it can be treated at home with an oral medicine.

Tuberculosis (TB)

TB is found in non-HIV-infected people as well as those with HIV, but people with HIV catch it much more easily and in a more severe form. TB is caused by *Mycobacterium tuberculosis*, a bacterium that mostly infects the lungs. But in some people with AIDS, TB can spread throughout the body. TB is particularly common in people who don't have good enough access to medical care. It causes cough, fever, and weight loss and spreads easily through the air around a person coughing out the TB bacteria. Fortunately, we can identify many people who have been exposed to TB by doing skin tests. People who are on effective treatment are no longer infectious to others. The treatment needed may be as many as four or more oral medicines, and it usually has to be given for a year or more. But staying on the TB medicine is very important, not only for the person with TB, but to protect other people.

Herpes Infections

There are two main types of herpes viruses, herpes simplex and herpes zoster. Herpes simplex type I causes sores (commonly known as cold sores) on the mouth and lips; herpes simplex type II causes sores on the genitals and anus. Sometimes herpes simplex can spread to other parts of the body. Herpes zoster is caused by the same virus that causes chickenpox. It often causes *shingles*, a painful rash that appears in one section of the skin. Again, in severe cases, herpes zoster can spread. Both types of herpes can affect people who don't have HIV, but they are often one of the early infections experienced by people with HIV. If the infection spreads to the eyes, it can be dangerous to the vision. There are medicines to treat some herpes infections, but others, like zoster, can be difficult to treat.

Cryptosporidiosis

In cryptosporidiosis, a parasite (*Cryptosporidium parvum*) infects the intestines and can cause diarrhea and cramping in the abdomen. The parasite is found in many animals and is passed on when food or water gets contaminated.

People with normal immune systems clear the parasite quite easily; those with a weak immune system may never clear it. Unfortunately, cryptosporidiosis is very difficult to treat. The most important task is to make sure that people with this disease don't get too dehydrated. Cryptosporidiosis and cryptococcosis are easy to mix up, but they're completely different.

Lymphoma

Lymphoma is a cancer of the lymph system caused by uncontrolled growth of abnormal lymph system cells. Most lymphoma in people with HIV is a type called non-Hodgkin's lymphoma. It can appear as fever, or night sweats with painless enlargement of a lymph node (gland) in one part of the body, when the lymph nodes in the other parts of the body aren't growing. It also can start in the brain and cause headaches, localized weakness, speech problems, or seizures. Non-Hodgkin's lymphoma is very difficult to treat. Chemotherapy is required and will sometimes shrink the tumor but rarely, if ever, completely cures it.

T Cells—T Helper Cells, CD4 Cells, and T4 Cells

Right now, the T cell count is the most useful of the tests available to monitor the effect of HIV on the immune system.

The T cell count is simply a blood test that measures the number of T helper cells (or CD4+ cells) in each cubic millimeter of blood. Because T cells are important in fighting infections and cancers, having a low T cell count increases the risk of illness. But T cell counts fluctuate quite a bit, even in healthy, HIV-negative people. All kinds of things affect the T cell count, such as stress, sleep, time of day, the lab where the test was done, and the presence of other infections. The T cell count is a bit like your blood pressure —it's important, but it goes up and down, and the trend is more important than any one reading.

Generally speaking, a T cell count between 500 and 1800 is normal for adults. A count between 200 and 500 indicates that the immune system is mildly suppressed, but people in this range are usually not at high risk for getting seriously ill. Most AIDS-associated diseases are rare when the T cell count is over 200. Kaposi's sarcoma (KS), tuberculosis (TB), and lymphoma are exceptions, but when a person's T cell count is over 200, these diseases appear in less dangerous forms. Problems such as oral candida (thrush) and skin problems can appear at this stage. Antiviral treatments such as AZT may be helpful.

A T cell count between 50 and 200 indicates that the immune system is more severely suppressed. Because of this, one of the definitions of AIDS includes any HIV-positive person with a T cell count less than 200. People with counts in this range definitely should take medication to prevent *Pneumocystis carinii* pneumonia (PCP) from developing and should strongly consider taking antiviral drugs. Many opportunistic infections (infections that develop when the immune system is weak but not when it's strong) develop when T cells are in this range. Nevertheless, lots of people with a T cell count less than 200 still feel healthy and may have no symptoms.

A T cell count below 50 indicates that the T cell part of the immune system is not functioning. Good, comprehensive medical care is vital, and treatment with medicines to prevent opportunistic infection is strongly recommended. Antiviral drugs such as AZT should be carefully considered, particularly for those who have never taken the drugs before. Most people who die of AIDS have a T cell count below 50. However, even at this low count, some people will feel well and have no AIDS-related problems. So T cells are important, but they're not the whole story.

Tests to measure blood levels of HIV have now been developed and may soon be in wide use. When we understand them better, these tests may allow us to choose anti-HIV medicines and do a better job of monitoring the immune system.

What Medications Are Available?

The main treatments used for HIV and AIDS are medications that act in one of four ways:

- *Antivirals* fight the HIV itself by preventing the HIV inside the body from reproducing. AZT, ddI, and ddC all act in this way.

- *Immune boosters* increase the body's immune response to invaders and to HIV itself. This approach may be promising for the future, but presently it is still experimental, and there are no approved treatments of this type. The therapeutic vaccines being developed are in this category. We will not be giving specific examples of medicines in this category, since all are experimental and there is not much reliable information about them.

- *Preventive medicines* prevent specific opportunistic infections. People with HIV are carefully monitored to find out when they are at high risk for certain specific diseases. Then if they move into a high-risk group, preventive medicines can be started. Preventive strategies for *Pneumocystis* and TB are well established. Now similar preventive strategies are being used or studied for MAC, toxoplasmosis, and CMV.

- *Treatment medicines* are used to treat specific opportunistic infections and diseases when they are identified.

In the following pages, we will discuss only a few of the more common medications used in HIV care. Much more extensive descriptions are widely available. Project Inform is one of the best resources (see "Suggested Reading" at the end of this chapter).

Antiviral Medications

Examples: The reverse transcriptase inhibitors are zidovudine (AZT, Retrovir),* didanosine (ddI, Videx), dideoxycytidine (ddC, Hivid), stavudine (d4T, Zerit), lamivudine (3TC, Epivir). A newer class of medications are the protease inhibitors: saquinavir, ritonavir, and indinavir.

How they work: Zidovudine, didanosine, dideoxycytidine, stavudine, and lamivudine inhibit a chemical called reverse transcriptase, which HIV uses to reproduce itself. HIV protease is a chemical that allows the HIV to make new, infectious virus particles. The protease inhibitors (saquinavir, ritonavir, and indinavir) keep the HIV protease from working, so that the HIV can't multiply.

Possible side effects: AZT often causes anemia (low red blood cell count) and neutropenia (low white blood cell count). AZT also can cause damage to the liver or the muscle tissue but does so rarely. Other common, but less serious, side effects include headaches, trouble sleeping, body aches, and nausea.

The drugs ddI, ddC, and d4T can cause neuropathy—tingling nerve pain that starts in the feet. In addition, ddI and ddC can cause inflammation of the pancreas, a potentially fatal (but rare) side effect. Diarrhea and stomach disturbances are common, but less serious, side effects.

3TC has few side effects, mainly nausea, vomiting, and headaches and rare cases of hair loss. Its major problem has been that it doesn't work well alone. It probably will be most useful in combination with AZT.

---

*Generic drug names are listed first, with alternate names for each drug in parentheses.

Saquinavir was well tolerated at all doses in one major study. But the protease inhibitors are very new—not much is known yet about the side effects that they could cause.

Comments: Until recently, antiviral drugs acting against the HIV reverse transcriptase were the only approved therapies for treating HIV infection. Now the protease inhibitors are coming into use, and it appears that this will be an important new class of drugs. Protease inhibitors will only be used in combination with reverse transcriptase inhibitors, however. And reverse transcriptase inhibitors still have been much more extensively tested than any other HIV drug. This means that although they have important side effects that can be severe, they also are a known quantity. They won't cause surprises, and if we're careful we can anticipate side effects and stop the drug early if they develop.

One of the major problems with this class of drugs is that HIV has shown an ability to develop resistance, often after a few years of therapy. A recent approach has been to treat with combination therapy. By combining AZT with one of the other four drugs, the chance of developing resistance can be reduced.

Preventive Medications

Using specific antibiotic medications to prevent opportunistic infections may be even more important than taking antiviral medicines.

Pneumocystis carinii Pneumonia (PCP)

Examples: Trimethoprim-sulfamethoxazole (Bactrim, Septra, TMP/SMX); aerosolized pentamidine (Nebupent, Aeropent); and dapsone. Atovaquone (Mepron, BW566) may be an appropriate preventive medication for a few people.

How they work: These medications all work by giving a steady low dose of antibiotic to kill *Pneumocystis* before there are enough organisms to create a true pneumonia.

Possible side effects: With TMP/SMX, the most common side effect is an allergic skin reaction resulting in rashes, which can be successfully managed. Fair-skinned people on TMP/SMX are also sensitive to sunlight. Other side effects include minor fevers, nausea, white count suppression, decreased platelet count, and liver irritation. Dapsone is associated with less severe occurrences of nausea, vomiting, rashes, lowered red and white cell counts, and liver dysfunction. People with low levels of G6PD (a liver function indicator) can develop rapid loss of blood cells on dapsone, so a G6PD test should be done before beginning dapsone treatment. The most common side effect of aerosolized pentamidine is a cough or raspy, dry throat, which can be minimized or eliminated by the use of inhaled medicines such as albuterol. Other side effects include a burning sensation in the back of the throat, an unpleasant taste, brief lung spasms, and (rarely) mild decrease in blood sugar. Atovaquone is well tolerated, but it is expensive and unproven in the setting of prevention.

Comments: TMP/SMX works extremely well for preventing PCP; almost no one who takes Septra regularly (daily or three times per week) comes down with the disease. The problem is that many people experience toxic reactions to TMP/SMX. These people should use one of the other medications.

Toxoplasmosis (Toxo)

Examples: Trimethoprim-sulfamethoxazole (Bactrim, Septra, TMP/SMX), dapsone, clindamycin, atovaquone (Mepron, BW566), and pyrimethamine have all been suggested for prevention of toxoplasmosis.

How they work: As with *Pneumocystis*, the idea is to kill the *Toxoplasma* organisms when they are present at a microscopic level, before they have started to invade brain tissue. The medications all work by giving a steady low dose of antibiotic. Steady low doses are particularly important for people with a low CD4 cell count and with a positive blood *Toxoplasma* antibody test (see Chapter 14).

Possible side effects: The side effects of TMP/SMX and dapsone (see *Pneumocystis* Pneumonia on page 193) are the same whether these drugs are for toxoplasmosis or *Pneumocystis* prevention. Atovaquone has fewer side effects. Clindamycin causes rash and/or diarrhea in many people. Pyrimethamine can cause loss of red blood cells in some people but is well tolerated in most.

Comments: People who need toxoplasmosis prevention almost always need *Pneumocystis* prevention too, so taking either TMP/SMX or dapsone can accomplish both goals. The other medications are less well proven but can be considered when a person is taking aerosolized pentamidine to prevent *Pneumocystis* and therefore needs another medicine to prevent toxoplasmosis.

Tuberculosis (TB)

Examples: Isoniazid (INH) is the most common medicine for preventing TB in people who have a positive skin test. Sometimes other drugs may be used if the doctor thinks you have been exposed to a resistant form of TB.

How they work: If you're around someone with TB, a small number of organisms may go into your lungs and create a tiny infection. This is enough to make your body react and make your skin test positive. INH, given for a year, can kill the infection before it becomes active.

Possible side effects: INH can occasionally cause liver disease. It can also cause neuropathy (nerve damage in the arms and legs), but this is easy to prevent by taking vitamin B6 while you're on the INH.

Comments: The skin test for TB is very important in order to catch TB before it becomes active. There is a big difference between taking one medication for preventing TB and waiting until the TB has spread, when usually at least four medications are needed.

Mycobacterium avium Complex (MAC)

Examples: Rifabutin, clarithromycin, and azithromycin are all effective for preventing MAC.

How they work: There is no blood or skin test for exposure to MAC, but we do know that the risk of MAC increases sharply when the CD4 cell count is below 100. If a person is at risk, taking rifabutin can cut the chances of getting MAC about in half. Like most of the prevention medicines, it works by killing the MAC before it has gotten a "foothold" in the body.

Possible side effects: Rifabutin can cause rashes, stomach upset, or a drop in the white blood cell count. However, most people tolerate it well.

Cytomegalovirus (CMV)

Examples: Only one medication, oral ganciclovir (Cytovene) is available for preventing CMV eye disease. Medicines to treat active CMV disease in the eyes or GI system (ganciclovir, foscarnet) must be given by vein (IV) or by central line (a special IV put in by the doctor that goes directly into the chest).

How they work: People at risk for CMV eye disease usually have been exposed to CMV before they get HIV. Oral ganciclovir works by "holding down" the spread of CMV to the eyes.

Possible side effects: Probably the biggest issue is that people on oral ganciclovir take 12 pills (!) per day, in addition to all the other medications they might be on. For many, this just seems like too much. Not surprisingly, some people have nausea and diarrhea. Ganciclovir can also cause decreased blood cell levels.

Comments: Using oral ganciclovir to prevent CMV retinitis is not yet a standard practice, but it is something to be considered.

Treatment Medications

Many of the medications we listed for preventing problems seen in HIV/ AIDS are also used for treating the problems when they occur. But treatment is always more difficult—it requires higher doses, more medicines, more complicated combinations, and it has more side effects. Many, many medications are used for treating different acute infections, and so we will not discuss all of them here. Generally speaking, all exert their toxic effects to kill the invading virus, bacteria, parasite, or fungus, and all attempt to do this with minimal toxicity to the cells of the human body. Your treatment team should be your first source for information about medicines used to treat acute infections, but there are other resources you can use, too. See the suggested reading and resources lists below.

Suggested Reading

Books

Project Inform. *The HIV Drug Book*. Old Tappan, NJ: Pocket Books, 1995. (An excellent and comprehensive HIV drug reference.)

Publications

AIDS Treatment News   (800) 873-2812
   (Biweekly reports on research, experimental
   therapies, and treatments)
BETA   (800) 959-1059
   (San Francisco AIDS Foundation quarterly)
Body Positive   (212) 566-7333
   (Nontechnical monthly magazine for
   HIV-positive people)
PI Perspectives   (800) 822-7422
   (Published by Project Inform with briefing
   papers issued between publications)
Positively Aware   (312) 472-6397
   (Published by the Test Positive Aware
   Network/Chicago)
Treatment Issues   (212) 337-3613
   (The GMHC newsletter of experimental therapies)

Resources

HIV/AIDS Treatment Information

Telephone Information

Centers for Disease Control (CDC) HIV/AIDS
    Treatment Information Service   (800) 448-0440

National Institutes of Health (NIH) AIDS
    Clinical Trials Information Service   (800) TRIALS-A

Project Inform Treatment Hotline   (800) 822-7422

World Wide Web Resources
(These change all the time, but are good places to start.)

Center for AIDS Prevention Studies
                          (http://chanane.ucsf.edu/capsweb/)

CDC National AIDS Clearinghouse Web Server
                (http://cdcnac.aspensys.com:86/nachome.html)

Marty Howard's HIV/AIDS HomePage
                          (http://www.smartlink.net/~martinjh/)

14

The Basic Prevention Panel

Most of the trouble people have with HIV is caused by opportunistic infections and cancers rather than by HIV itself. In theory, if we could prevent these opportunistic infections and cancers from happening, people with HIV/AIDS could do quite well. A lot of the routine care that is helpful for people with HIV is meant to prevent, rather than cure, health problems. It is much better to prevent diseases than to wait for them to happen.

Four strategies will help you prevent disease:

- Strengthen the immune system against infections with antivirals and immunizations.

- Eliminate traces of infection with preventive antibiotics before the infection develops into disease.

- Detect signs of infection early, so it can be treated before it causes problems.

- Adopt appropriate lifestyle changes that promote or maintain general good health.

To make sure you're getting the best care possible, you need to make sure you stay up to date on your basic prevention panel. The tables on the next few pages list the basic tests, medications, and vaccines that we recommend for adults with HIV/AIDS (children are different—don't use these guidelines for them). Remember that these are basic guidelines. For most people, these guidelines act as a minimum standard, but many doctors and people with HIV/AIDS will do more than what is listed here. You and your doctor might decide to do things differently, given special circumstances. But if you decide *not* to do one or more of the things listed, it should be because you've thought about it, talked to your doctor about it, and made an informed and careful decision. That's the essence of being a self-manager.

To use the tables, look under the correct table for your T cell count* and make sure that you and your doctor do each of the things listed. Prepare by making a list to bring to the doctor's office.

---

*We discuss T cells and the meaning of the various T cell counts in Chapter 13.

Soon After You Test Positive for HIV (Any T Cell Count)

Tests	Medications	Vaccines	Self-Care
Skin test for TB[1] (PPD[2] tuberculin test) and skin test for anergy[3]	Isoniazid (INH) therapy for one year *if* PPD test positive *and* no active TB		Find a good provider whom you like and who knows about HIV.
Complete blood count (white blood cell levels, red blood cell levels, anemia, platelets)		Diphtheria-tetanus (every 10 years)	
T cell count (absolute T helper cell count and percent T helper cell count)		Pneumococcal vaccine (once)	
Baseline syphilis blood test		Influenza vaccine (every fall)	
Baseline hepatitis B blood test		Hepatitis B vaccine if the hepatitis B blood test is negative (series of 3 shots once)	
Toxoplasmosis antibody test			
Baseline chest X ray			
Baseline vaginal exam and Pap smear test (women)			Time to think hard about changing your health habits: safer sex, smoking, alcohol, drugs.
Baseline oral/ dental exam			
Baseline neurological exam			

[1] Tuberculosis
[2] Purified Protein Derivative (used in skin tests for tuberculosis)
[3] Anergy skin testing checks to make sure your immune system can respond to skin tests.

T Cell Count > 600

Tests	Medications	Vaccines	Self-Care
Skin test for TB (PPD tuberculin test) and skin test for anergy every 6 months	Isoniazid (INH) therapy for one year *if* PPD test positive *and* no active TB		Now is the time to start educating yourself about treatment options.
T cell count (absolute T helper cell count and percent T helper cell count) every 6 months		Influenza vaccine (every fall)	
Syphilis blood test every year or after any possible sexual exposure			
Prompt exam by eye doctor if vision problems develop			Use the Amsler grid to monitor vision.*
Hepatitis B blood test every year or after any possible new exposure			
Vaginal exam and Pap smear test (women) every 6–12 months			
Oral/dental exam every 6 months			

*See Chapter 17, "Helpful Hints."

T Cell Count 200–600			
Tests	Medications	Vaccines	Self-Care
Skin test for TB (PPD tuberculin test) and skin test for anergy every 6 months	Isoniazid (INH) therapy for one year *if* PPD test positive *and* no active TB		
T cell count (absolute T helper cell count and percent T helper cell count) every 3 months	*If T cell count is < 500,* you and your doctor should discuss starting antiretroviral therapy.*	Influenza vaccine (every fall)	Build a partnership with your doctor. You may also want to think about being in a drug trial.
Syphilis blood test every year or after any possible sexual exposure			
Prompt exam by eye doctor if vision problems develop			Use the Amsler grid to monitor vision.**
Hepatitis B blood test every year or after any possible new exposure			
Vaginal exam and Pap smear test (women) every 6–12 months			
Oral/dental exam every 6 months			Don't forget about exercise and good nutrition.

*Antiretroviral therapy is therapy with medications that attack the HIV itself.
**See Chapter 17, "Helpful Hints."

T Cell Count 100–200

Tests	Medications	Vaccines	Self-Care
Skin test for TB (PPD tuberculin test) and skin test for anergy every 6 months	Isoniazid (INH) therapy for one year *if* PPD test positive *and* no active TB		Make sure you know about your doctor's night/weekend coverage in case you need it.
T cell count (absolute T helper cell count and percent T helper cell count) every 3 months	*Start a medication for preventing* Pneumocystis *(PCP) (Septra, dapsone, or inhaled pentamidine).*	Influenza vaccine (every fall)	Build a partnership with your doctor. You may also want to think about being in a drug trial.
Syphilis blood test every year or after any possible sexual exposure	You and your doctor should discuss starting antiretroviral therapy, or if you have already been on an antiretroviral, discuss switching.		
Prompt exam by eye doctor if vision problems develop			Use the Amsler grid to monitor vision.*
Hepatitis B blood test every year or after any possible new exposure			Nutrition and exercise are very important. Liquid supplements may help if you're losing weight.
Vaginal exam and Pap smear test (women) every 6–12 months			
Oral/dental exam every 6 months			

*See Chapter 17, "Helpful Hints."

T Cell Count < 100

Tests	Medications	Vaccines	Self-Care
Skin test for TB (PPD tuberculin test) and skin test for anergy every 6 months	Isoniazid (INH) therapy for one year *if* PPD test positive *and* no active TB		Make sure you know about your doctor's night/ weekend coverage in case you need it.
T cell count as needed to aid diagnosis or treatment decisions	*Continue regular medications for preventing Pneumocystis (PCP) (Septra, dapsone, inhaled pentamidine)*	Influenza vaccine (every fall)	
Syphilis blood test every year or after any possible sexual exposure	You and your doctor should discuss starting medication for preventing MAC.		
Baseline eye exam by eye doctor. Repeat at least every year or if vision problems develop.	You and your doctor should discuss switching antiretroviral medications.		Use the Amsler grid to monitor vision.*
Hepatitis B blood test every year or after any possible new exposure			Nutrition and exercise are very important. Liquid supplements may help if you're losing weight.
Vaginal exam and Pap smear test (women) every 6–12 months			
Oral/dental exam every 6 months			

*See Chapter 17, "Helpful Hints."

Suggested Reading

Managing Early HIV Infection. AHCPR Publication No. 94-0573. Rockville, MD: U.S. Department of Health and Human Services, 1994.

Martelli, Leonard J., et al. *When Someone You Know Has AIDS: A Practical Guide.* New York: Crown, 1993.

Petrow, Steven (ed). *The HIV Drug Book.* New York: Pocket Books, 1995. (The only reference available that lists and describes all the drugs used by people with HIV, their effects, and their interactions.)

Schwartz, Ruth. *AIDS Medical Guide.* San Francisco: San Francisco AIDS Foundation, 1992.

PART 5

Managing
Practical Details

15

Planning for the Future—
Fears and Reality

This book is about living well with HIV/AIDS by taking charge of day-to-day problems and challenges and coming up with ways to solve them. Whether your problem is getting used to a new medicine, starting a new exercise routine, or dealing with the death of someone you love, the principles are the same. In this chapter we discuss some of the big questions people often have trouble thinking about. These questions tend to be about all the "big unmentionables" in life: becoming dependent, money issues, sex, grief, and death. We touch on all of them and give some suggestions that you may find useful.

The future can be frightening for people with chronic illness. The most common way that people deal with their fear about the future is that they *don't* deal with it. People with illnesses often put off doing or thinking anything about the future, because they think it will be too depressing or that there's nothing they can do to make any difference. Of course, if you *think* that nothing you do will make a difference, then you probably won't do anything, and your prediction will come true. There are so many things to be concerned about—disability, loss of independence, money problems, even death.

What if I Can't Take Care
of Myself Anymore?

Becoming helpless and dependent is the most basic fear among people who have a potentially disabling health problem. This fear usually has physical, as well as financial, social, and emotional components.

Physical Concerns of Day-to-Day Living

As your health condition changes over time, you may need to consider changing your living situation. Change may involve hiring someone to help you in your home or moving to a living situation where help is provided. The decision about which alternative is best will be related to your needs and how they can best be met.

The first thing you will need to do is carefully *evaluate what you can do for yourself,* and what activities of daily living (ADLs) will require some kind of help. ADLs are the everyday things like getting out of bed, bathing, dressing, preparing and eating your meals, cleaning house, shopping, paying bills, and so forth. Most people can do all of these, even though they may have to do them slowly, with some modification, or with some help from gadgets.

Some people, though, may eventually find one or more of these ADLs no longer possible without help from somebody else. For example, you may still be able to fix meals, but your mobility may be impaired to the degree that shopping is no longer possible. Or, if you have problems with fainting or sudden bouts of unconsciousness, you might need to have somebody around at all times.

When you have analyzed your situation, you should make a list, with one column for those activities that you need help with, and the other column for some ideas on what kind of help you might look for. For example:

Need Help With	*What Kind of Help to Look For*
Can't go shopping	• Get friend to shop for me
	• Find volunteer shopping service
	• Shop at store that delivers
	• Ask neighbor to shop for me when she does her own shopping
	• Get home-delivered meals
Can't be by myself	• Hire around-the-clock attendant
	• Move in with a relative
	• Get a "life-line" emergency response system
	• Move to board and care home
	• Move into shared-housing community or group home for people with HIV/AIDS

When you have listed your problems, and their possible solutions, select the solution that seems the most workable, acceptable, and least expensive for your needs.

The selection should depend upon your finances, the family or other resources you can call on, and how well any of the potential solutions will in fact solve your problem. Sometimes one solution will be the answer for several problems. For instance, if you can't shop, can't be alone, and maybe household chores are reaching the point of a foreseeable need for help, you might consider that an assisted-living environment or group home will solve all these problems, since it offers assistance with meals, regular house cleaning, and transportation for errands and medical appointments.

Even if you are not of "retirement" age, many facilities accept younger people, depending on the facility's particular policies. Most facilities for the retired take residents as young as 50, or younger if one of a couple is the minimum age. If you are a young person, the local center for the disabled or independent living center should be able to direct you to an out-of-home care facility that is appropriate for you.

Your appraisal of your situation and needs may well be aided by sitting down with a trusted friend or relative and discussing your abilities and limitations. Sometimes another person can spot things that we ourselves overlook, or would like to ignore.

Make changes in your life slowly, incrementally. You don't need to change your whole life around to solve one problem. Remember, too, that you can always change your mind, if you don't "burn your bridges behind you." If you think that moving out of your own place to another living arrangement (relatives, care home, and so on) would be the thing to do, don't give up your present home until you are settled in to your new home and are sure you want to stay there. If you think you need help with some activities, hiring help at home is less drastic than moving out, and may be enough for quite a while. If you can't be alone, and you live with a family member who is away from home during the day, maybe going to an adult or senior day care center will be enough to keep you safe and comfortable while your family is away. In fact, adult day care centers are ideal places to find new friends and activities geared to your abilities.

There are several kinds of professionals who can be of great help in giving you ideas about how to deal with your care needs:

- *A social worker* at your AIDS organization, center for the disabled, or your hospital social services department can be very helpful in helping you decide how to solve financial and living arrangement problems and locating appropriate community resources. Some social workers are also trained in counseling the disabled in relation to emotional and relationship problems that may be associated with your health problem.

- *A licensed occupational therapist* can assess your daily living needs and suggest assistive devices or rearrangements in your environment to make life easier.

- *An attorney* should be on your "must see" list to help you set your financial affairs in order to preserve your assets, to prepare a proper will, and perhaps to execute a durable power of attorney for both health care and financial management. If finances are a concern, ask your local AIDS organization for the names of attorneys who offer free or low-cost services. Your local bar association or legal aid office can also refer you to a list of attorneys who are competent in this area.

Finding In-Home Help

If you find that you cannot manage your ADLs alone, your first option is usually to hire somebody to help. Most people just need a person called a *home aide*, or some similar title. Home aides provide no medically related services needing special licensing, but do help with bathing, dressing, meal preparation, and household chores.

You can find in-home help in a number of ways:

- *Home care agencies* are the easiest, but most expensive, way to find home care. You will usually find them listed under "home care" or "home nursing" in the telephone directory yellow pages. Such agencies are usually (but not always) private, for-profit businesses that supply caregiver staff to private individuals at home. The fees charged vary with the skill and license of the caregiver and will include an amount for Social Security, insurance, bonding, and profit for the agency. The fees are usually about double what you would expect to pay for someone you hire directly. The advantage, if you can afford it, is that the agency assumes all payroll responsibilities, including Social Security and federal and state taxes, responsibility for the skill and integrity of the attendant, and immediate replacement of an ill or no-show attendant. The agency pays the staff directly. The client has no involvement with paying the attendant, but pays the agency.

- *Registered nurses* (R.N.'s) hired this way are very expensive, but it is rare that home care for a chronically ill person requires a registered nurse.

Licensed vocational nurses (L.V.N.'s) will cost somewhat less, but are still expensive, and are usually not needed unless there are nursing services required (such as dressing changes, injections, ventilator management, and so forth). *Certified Nursing Assistants* (C.N.A.'s) have some basic training in nursing, are much less expensive, and can provide satisfactory care for all but the most critically ill person at home. Most of these agencies also supply *home aides* as well as licensed staff. Unless you are bed-ridden or require some procedure that must be done by someone with a certain category of license, a home aide will probably be the most appropriate for your needs.

- *Registries* supply prescreened lists of attendants or caregivers from which you select the one you wish to hire. You will be charged a placement fee, usually equal to one month's pay of the person hired. The agency will assume no liability for the skill or honesty of the people on its list, and you will need to check references and interview carefully, just as you would someone who comes from any other source. This type of resource can be found in the yellow pages under the same listing as "home nursing agencies" or "registries." Some agencies provide both their own staff and registries of staff for you to select from.

- *Senior centers and centers serving the disabled population* may also provide home help. They often have listings of people who have called them to say they want work as a home attendant or who have put a notice up on a bulletin board there. These job seekers are not screened; you will need to interview them carefully and check their references before hiring someone.

- *The classified "employment wanted" section of your local newspaper* can also be a good resource for experienced home care attendants. Since their patients usually progress to a need for more or sometimes less care than home attendants provide, their jobs are by nature temporary and they often must look for new work. You can find a competent helper through the newspaper, but the advice to interview carefully is valid here, too.

- *Word of mouth* is probably your best source of help. Look for someone who has employed a person, or knows of somebody who has worked for someone they know. Putting the word out through your family and social network may result in a jewel.

- *Home sharing* may be a solution if you have space and could offer a home to someone in exchange for help. This arrangement works best if you need help mainly with household and garden chores. However, some people may be willing to provide personal care, such as help with dressing and bathing and meal preparation. Some communities have agencies or government bureaus that help home-sharers and home-sharees locate each other.

Finding Out-of-Home Care

If getting the care you need just isn't possible in your own home, it may be time to think about moving somewhere where you can be safe and comfortable. Here are some of the options to look into.

Residential Care Homes

Residential care homes, or *board and care homes*, are licensed by the state or county social services agency. They provide nonmedical care and supervision for persons who cannot live alone. These homes fall into two categories: large and small. The small ones have about six "residents," who live in a family-like setting in a neighborhood residence. The large ones have more residents, sometimes hundreds, who live in a boarding house or hotel-like setting. They take meals in a central dining room and have individual or shared rooms, with activities in large common rooms.

In either type of facility, the services to the residents are the same—all meals, assistance with bathing and dressing as needed, laundry, housekeeping, transportation to medical appointments, supervision, and assistance with taking medications. In the larger facilities, there are usually professional activities directors. Residents of the larger facilities usually need to be more independent, since there tends not to be as much personal attention as is provided by the smaller homes.

These homes are licensed in most states for either "elderly" (over 62) or "adult" (under 62). The adult category is further divided into facilities for mentally ill, mentally retarded, or physically disabled.

It is important when considering a residential care home to evaluate the type of persons who are already living there to make sure that you will fit in. For example, some of these facilities may cater to individuals who are mentally confused. If you are mentally clear, you would not find much companionship there. If everyone is hard of hearing, you might find conversation tiring.

Although all homes are by law required to provide wholesome meals, you should make sure the cuisine is to your liking and can meet your dietary needs. If you need a vegetarian or diabetic diet, for instance, be sure the operator is willing to prepare your special diet.

The monthly fees for residential care homes vary, depending upon whether they are spartan or luxurious. The most spartan facilities cost about the same as the SSI (Supplemental Security Income) benefit and will take SSI beneficiaries, billing the government directly. The more luxurious the home is with respect to furnishings, neighborhood, services, and so on, the greater the cost. Even the nicest of these will probably cost less than full-time, 24-hour, 7-day at-home care.

Skilled Nursing Facilities

Sometimes called *nursing homes* or *convalescent hospitals,* the *skilled nursing facility* provides the most comprehensive care for severely ill or disabled people. If you have PCP or toxoplasmosis, you may need to be transferred from an acute hospital to a skilled nursing facility for a period of rehabilitation before going home.

No care situation seems to inspire more fear than the prospect of having to go to a nursing home. "Horror stories" in the news media help to foster the anxiety about what awful fate will befall anyone who has the misfortune to have to go there. However, public scrutiny is valuable in helping assure that standards of care and humane and competent treatment are provided. It must be remembered that nursing homes serve a critical need. When you really need a nursing home, usually no other care situation will meet this need.

Skilled nursing facilities provide medically related care for people who are no longer able to be in a nonmedical care situation. For example, you may need to have intravenous or injected medications that must be administered or monitored by professional nursing staff. Or you may be very physically limited, needing to have help with getting in and out of bed, eating, bathing, or dealing with bladder or bowel control. Skilled nursing facilities can also manage care of feeding tubes, respirators, and other high-tech care equipment. If you are only partially or temporarily disabled, you may need a skilled nursing facility for physical, occupational, and speech therapy; wound care; or other therapies.

Not all nursing homes provide all types of care. Some specialize in rehabilitation and therapies, and some specialize in long-term, custodial care. Some are able to provide high-tech nursing services; others do not.

In selecting a nursing home, you should seek out the help of the *hospital discharge planner* or *social worker,* or a similar professional from a home care agency or center for the disabled. There are organizations to monitor local nursing homes. Each nursing home is required by law to post in a prominent place the name and phone number of the "ombudsman," a person assigned by the state licensing agency to assist patients and their families with problems in relation to their nursing home care. The agencies that can help you with this are listed in the yellow pages under "social service organizations."

Hospice

Hospice care is an important option that, although it isn't for everyone, everyone should at least know about. Hospice philosophy is based on the belief that death is part of life and is something that we will all experience. Therefore, hospice care concentrates on relieving pain and supporting emotional and spiritual needs. Hospice care doesn't emphasize prolonging life as long as is medically possible. Instead, the individual is given an environment to reflect on life and develop a sense of peace. The hope is that with good hospice care, a person can meet the end more peacefully than might otherwise be possible.

Many communities have excellent hospice facilities where people with serious illnesses can live and be cared for during the final stage of life. Good hospice care can often be done in your own home, too. The best way to find out about hospice care is through your local AIDS service organization or through your medical care site.

Will I Have Enough Money to Pay for My Care?

Next to the basic fear of physical dependency, the greatest fear of most people with serious illness is not having enough money to pay for their needs. Being sick often requires care and treatment that is expensive. If you are too ill or disabled to work, the loss of income, and especially your health insurance coverage, may present an overwhelming financial burden. You can, however, avoid some of the risks by planning ahead and knowing your resources. There are a number of government benefit programs you should know about.

- *Social Security.* If you are too sick to work—either permanently, or for some extended period—you may be entitled to draw Social Security on the basis of your disability. People with symptomatic HIV infection may be able to document their disability simply by showing they have had one or more illnesses—such as *Pneumocystis* pneumonia (PCP), toxoplasmosis, HIV wasting syndrome, and others—that lead to "automatic" disability. People who haven't had one of these illnesses may have to get other documentation that they qualify. If you qualify and have dependent children, they would also receive Social Security bene-fits. If you have been disabled for a specified period (as of this writing, it is two years) you may be entitled to Medicare coverage for your medical treatment needs.

- *Medicaid and SSI.* If you have only minimal savings and little or no income, the federal Medicaid program can pay for medical treatment and long-term skilled or custodial care. The eligibility rules on assets and income differ from state to state. If you have savings of less than the U.S. median of one month's wages, and income at or slightly above the official federal "poverty line" (this changes from year to year), you should consult your local social services department to see if you are entitled to benefits. If Social Security benefits are unavailable or insuffi-cient, the Supplemental Security Income (SSI) program is available to those who meet the same eligibility criteria as for Medicaid.

  The SSI and the Medicaid programs are available to those who have little or no income or savings. If you have some savings, you will have to pay for your care until you have "spent down" to meet the asset limi-tation criteria. If you have income above a certain level, you will have what is termed a "co-payment," or "share-of-cost," which you must pay before Medicaid would begin to supplement.

The social work department in the hospital where you have obtained treatment can advise you about your own situation and the probability of your being eligible for these programs. The local agency serving the disabled also usually has benefits counselors or advisors who can refer you to programs and resources for which you may be eligible. Your local AIDS and community service organizations often have benefit counselors who are knowledgeable about the ins-and-outs of health care insurance.

Be warned: Although the government can provide a helpful (and in some cases lifesaving) safety net, dealing with government agencies is difficult. Be patient, expect problems, and keep at it.

I Need Help, But I Don't Want Help. Now What?

We all emerge from childhood reaching for and cherishing every possible sign of independence—the driver's license, the first job, the first checking account, the first time we go out and don't have to tell anyone where we are going or when we will be back, and so on. In these, and many other ways, we demonstrate to ourselves as well as to others that we are in charge of our lives and able to take care of ourselves without any help from parents.

If a time comes when we must face the realization that we need help, that we can no longer manage completely on our own, it may seem like a return to childhood and having to let somebody else be in charge of our lives. This dependency can be very painful and embarrassing. Some people in this situation become extremely depressed and can no longer find any joy in life. Others fight off the recognition of their need for help, thus placing themselves in possible danger and making life difficult and frustrating for those who would like to be helpful. Some people give up completely and expect others to take total responsibility for their lives, demanding attention and services from their partners, friends, and family. If you are having one or more of these reactions, you can help yourself feel better and develop a more positive response.

"Let me have the courage to change the things I can change, to accept the things I cannot change, and to have the wisdom to know the difference." This concept is fundamental to staying in charge of your life. You must be able to correctly evaluate your situation. You must identify those activities that require the help of somebody else (going shopping or cleaning house, for instance) and those activities you can still do on your own (getting dressed, paying bills, writing letters). This means making decisions, and as long as you keep the decisionmaking prerogative, you are in charge. It is important to make a decision and take action while you are still able to do so, before circumstances intervene and the decision gets made for you. That means being realistic and honest with yourself.

There are several proactive approaches you can take to get help and still stay in charge of your life:

- *Talk with a sympathetic listener,* either a professional counselor or a sensible, close friend or family member. An objective listener often helps by pointing out alternatives and options that you may have overlooked or were not aware of. Such a person can provide information or another point of view or interpretation of a situation that you would not have come upon yourself. This is part of the self-management process. Be very careful however, in evaluating advice from someone who has something to sell you. There are many people whose solution to your problem just happens to be whatever it is they are selling—health or burial insurance policies, special furniture, "sunshine cruises," special magazines, or health foods with curative properties.

- *Be as open and reasonable as you can be* when talking with family members or friends who offer to be helpful, yet at the same time, try to make them understand that you will reserve for yourself the right to decide how much and what kind of help you will accept. They will probably be more cooperative and understanding if you can say, "Yes, I do need some help with . . . , but I still want to do . . . myself."

- *Insist on being consulted.* Lay the ground rules with your helpers early on. Ask to be presented with choices, so that you can decide what is best for you as you see it. If you try to objectively weigh the suggestions made to you and don't dismiss every option out of hand, people will consider you able to make reasonable decisions and will continue to provide you the opportunity to do so.

- *Be appreciative.* Recognize the good will and the efforts of those who want to help. Even though you may be embarrassed, you will maintain your dignity by accepting with grace the help that is offered, if you need it. If you are truly convinced that you are being offered help you don't need, you can decline it with tact and appreciation. For example, you can say, "I appreciate your offer to have Thanksgiving at your house, but I'd like to continue having it here. I could really use some help, though—maybe with the clean-up after dinner."

- *Consult a professional counselor* if you are at length unable to come to terms with your increasing need to be dependent upon others for help in managing your living situation. This should be someone who has experience with the emotional and social issues of people with disabling health problems. Your local agency providing services to the disabled should be able to refer you to the right kind of counselor. The local or national organization dedicated to serving people with HIV/AIDS can also refer you to support groups and classes to help you in dealing with your condition. You should be able to locate the agency you need through the telephone book yellow pages under the listing "social service organizations."

We need to be sure that we do reach out to family and friends and ask for the help we need when we recognize that we can't go on alone. It sometimes happens that, expecting rejection, people fail to ask for help. Some people try to hide their need in fear that their need will cause loved ones to withdraw. Families often complain, "If we'd only known . . . ," when it is revealed that a loved one had needs for help that were unmet.

If you really cannot turn to close family or friends because they are unable or unwilling to become involved in your care, there are agencies which are dedicated to providing for such situations. Through your local social service department's "adult protective services" program or Family Services Association you should be able to locate a "case manager" who will be able to organize the resources in your community to provide the help you need. The social services department in your local hospital can also put you in touch with the right agency.

Does My Illness Mean an End to Sex?

Having HIV/AIDS should not redefine a person as an asexual being who's lost interest in sex. If anything, a person who has to face and adapt to changes caused by a chronic disease needs the love and comfort of a close, intimate relationship perhaps more than ever. However, this aspect of life is often ignored, denied, or feared. For one thing, people with HIV/AIDS are rightly concerned about the risk that they will spread HIV to others. Learning to practice safer sex is necessary, but it's hard, and sometimes it seems easier just not to bother. Some people worry that the strenuousness of sex will make them weaker. Sometimes HIV/AIDS itself can lead to changes in hormone levels and therefore decreased sex drive. People with breathing difficulties worry that sex is too strenuous and will bring on an attack of coughing and wheezing, or worse.

One of the most subtle and devastating barriers to fulfilling sexuality is the damage that HIV/AIDS may cause to your self-image and self-esteem. You may believe you are physically unattractive as a result of your disease—for example, because of paralysis, shortness of breath, weight loss from medication, or a sense of not being really a whole, functioning being. This may cause you to avoid sexual situations, and you may "try not to think about it."

Attitude and communication are the keys to resuming the sexual aspect of your relationships. You must believe that sex is a necessary and rewarding part of your life, and you must communicate that to your partner.

As of this writing there are few instructional materials on sexuality specifically written for physically disabled people. There are, however, a number of very useful general how-to guides in the bookstores for those wanting to enhance their sexual relationships. If you understand and appreciate your own needs and preferences, and those of your partner, you can use creativity in adapting the activities described in these guides to your own relationship. It is important to avoid any assumptions that there is only one "right way" to be sexually fulfilled.

Here are some ways to help you enhance sexual fulfillment:

- *Talk about your HIV status.* Your partner needs to know, and the sooner you do it, the sooner you can move on to healthy, enjoyable safer sex practices.

- *Try to establish a calm and relaxed atmosphere.* Stressful or highly emotional conversations tend to cause anxiety and are not conducive to satisfying sexual activities.

- *Find positions that are comfortable* for both of you. Try to achieve open communication with your partner about what you like and want in the course of sexual activities.

- *Avoid sexual activity when you feel really tired.*

- *Avoid sexual activity right after a big meal.*

- *Avoid drinking alcohol before sex.*

- If you have trouble with sexual performance, *check with your doctor to see if you are taking medication that may be the cause.* Adjustments in dosage or switching to another medication may help.

- *Keep physically fit.* Being fit enhances sexual performance.

- *Enjoy a romantic weekend.* Special "marriage encounter" weekends are available through some churches for people who want to enhance their marriages in general. Gay couples can get help with planning weekends from a travel agent that specifically caters to the gay community.

- *Consult a professional experienced in sexual counseling* if you are having chronic problems with arousal, or a chronic loss of interest in sex. Short-term problems are often due to depression.

Grieving—A Normal Reaction to Bad News

When we experience any kind of a loss—small (such as losing a favorite possession), or large (such as losing a life partner or facing a disabling or terminal illness)—we go through an emotional process of grieving and coming to terms with the loss. A person with a chronic, disabling health problem experiences a variety of losses—loss of confidence, loss of self-esteem, loss of independence, loss of lifestyle, and perhaps the most painful of all, the loss of positive self-image if the condition has an effect on personal appearance.

Elisabeth Kübler-Ross, who has written extensively about this process, describes the stages of grief as:

- *Shock*, when we feel both a mental and a physical reaction to the initial recognition of the loss
- *Denial*, when we tell ourself, "No, it can't be true," and proceed to act for a time as if it were not true
- *Anger*, when we ask, "Why me?" and search for someone or something to blame ("If the doctor had diagnosed it early enough, I'd have been cured," or "The job caused me too much stress," and so on).
- *Bargaining*, when we say to ourself, to someone else, to God, "I'll never smoke again . . . ," or "I'll follow my treatment regimen absolutely to the letter . . . ," or "I'll go to church every Sunday . . . ," ". . . if only I can get over this."
- *Depression*, when the real awareness sets in, we really confront the truth about the situation, and experience deep feelings of sadness and hopelessness.
- *Acceptance*, when we eventually recognize that we must deal with what has happened, and make up our minds to do what we have to do.

We do not pass through these stages in a linear out-of-one-and-into-the-next fashion. We are more apt to have several, or even many, flip-flops back and forth between them. Don't be discouraged if you find yourself angry or depressed again just when you thought you had reached acceptance. Many people get stuck at the depression stage of the grief process; however, as we discussed in Chapter 4, there are several ways for you to move out of this stage toward acceptance.

Recognizing Depression

As discussed in Chapter 4, the most consistent and significant core element in depression is a *sense of powerlessness*. This is perceived as feeling helpless and unable to restore one's losses or to have any effect on events or their outcome. We find it appropriate to review and amplify our discussion of depression here.

People may sometimes hide their depression from themselves because they cannot bring themselves to face and deal with their unhappy situation and the implications for their future. Instead, they often express depression in behavioral ways. It is not uncommon for people who are experiencing a reactive depression to find themselves *sleeping a lot* or unable to sleep well, *overeating* or not hungry at all, *avoiding people* and places they used to find interesting, or finding that they *cannot stand to be alone*, even for a little while.

Increased irritability or impatience are typical ways to express depression, though these outbursts are often unrelated to real events, often mystifying the person who is the target of one's irascibility. Sudden *neglect of personal appearance* or business or personal concerns is not uncommon in a depressed person. Depressed people often find themselves unable to enjoy activities, experiences, or relationships that previously were satisfying.

Not all depression behavior is negative. Sometimes *unrealistic "cheeriness"* will mask what the person is really feeling, and the wise observer will recognize the brittleness or phoniness of the mood. *Refusal to accept offers of help*, even in the face of obvious need for it, is a frequent symptom of unrecognized depression.

Depression behavior tends to be excessive in one direction or another from what would be considered normal for that individual.

The paradox of depression behavior is that the more one engages in the behavior the more likely one will ultimately drive away the people who are most able to provide the comfort and support that the depressed person needs in their time of sorrow. Most of our friends and family want to help us feel better, but often they don't really know what to do to help. As their efforts to comfort and reassure us are frustrated, they may at some point throw up their hands and quit trying. Then the depressed person winds up saying, "See, nobody cares," thus reinforcing the feelings of loss and loneliness.

What to Do About Depression

The first thing to do is to *recognize* that you may be depressed then to take action aimed to reverse the feelings. If you perceive depression in yourself, or hear associates complaining that you are exhibiting behaviors described above, stop and take stock. Consider that your nearest and dearest may be telling you the truth.

There are several different ways to manage depression, and probably the most direct and effective approach is to take steps to restore your sense of self-worth and autonomy. If you can *begin to take charge* of your situation, you will begin to feel stronger and more effective and to develop a sense of personal power. This means that you must be willing to make the decisions you can make, do for yourself what you can actually do, and engage in the problem-solving self-management process.

It is important that you *develop the ability to communicate* your needs and thoughts effectively. If your loved ones want to help you it will help them to have you tell them how they can best do that. As discussed in Chapter 10, a candid assessment of your needs, and the simple and direct statement to another person about how they can help will keep you in the autonomous position. If you can say, "Could you pick up some groceries for me while you are at the store?" it will keep another from having to guess (often wrongly) at what you need, and give them a sense of importance at being able to help you. Most people love to feel important to another person and are grateful for the opportunity. The only catch is not to overdo to the point of becoming a burden. "Please, could you open the door for me?" is more dignified than struggling with the door while an onlooker stands by feeling uncomfortable about your predicament, not knowing whether or not to offer to help.

As you become aware of your needs for help and as these needs increase, it will be important to *sit down with those closest to you and share* with them what is happening to you, and the implications with respect to your abilities and limitations. You will need to provide them with an honest representation of how your condition will affect them and to evaluate realistically what kind of help you will be needing and how that help might be best provided. If you will soon be unable to pursue an activity, such as square dancing or tennis, or perform some task, such as driving the car, those who will be affected need to know. They will also need to be reassured that you will still be able to do many things, and that even though, for instance, you no longer play golf, you would love to play cards or go to concerts, instead. Your loved ones also need to know that you intend to remain as functional as possible, both physically and mentally, and that you don't want to be considered totally helpless, even though you do have limitations.

As you can see, *communication with others* is a key part of dealing with your depressed state of mind. Techniques for effective communication are discussed in Chapter 10 in this book.

Many depressed people isolate themselves at home and endure their misery alone. Though the idea may at first seem unappealing, if you have been avoiding company, do make opportunities to *be among people*, even if only by a telephone call to a friend, or having somebody come over for coffee or a meal. When you are with somebody, resist the inclination to discuss your medical condition and how you feel about it and instead focus on what is going on in the life of the person you are with.

Distraction and intellectual stimulation will help you feel better and divert your focus from yourself and your problems to things outside yourself. Your favorite music or other entertainment, enjoyed in the company of a friend or family member can raise your spirits. Joining a group or class that is learning a new skill will feed your need to feel more capable. Research about your condition and treatments will make you a better treatment team partner with your doctor and better prepared to take charge of your treatment decisions.

Practice positive "self-talk." Scientific research has proven that positive thinking is very highly associated with positive outcomes. The human mind's ability to affect the body is truly miraculous. It is almost impossible to feel sad when we say something happy. The power of "I think I can do it" to enable us to accomplish is enormous. This phenomenon is called "self-efficacy." Self-talk can be a very effective way to gain control of your emotions and attitudes. When you feel depressed, practicing positive, optimistic thoughts, in the form of the internal conversations that you hold with yourself will help you feel better emotionally and physically.

"Feelings are facts" is a way of saying that what we feel is real to us, regardless of whether or not the feelings are realistic. What we do about these feelings depends upon our attitude—about ourselves, about our ability to solve our problems, about the prospects of a satisfying life. If our attitude is positive and goal oriented, if we believe that we can still make some good things happen in our lives, then we will be able to do that. There is magic in believing.

I'm Afraid of Death

Fear of death is something most of us only begin to experience when something happens to bring us face-to-face with the possibility of our own death. Losing someone close, an accident that might have been fatal, or learning we have a health condition that may shorten our lives usually causes us to consider the inevitability of our own eventual passing. Many people, even then, try to avoid facing the future because they are afraid to think about it.

If you are ready to think about your own future—about the near or distant prospect that your life will most certainly end at some time—then the ideas that follow will be useful to you. If you are not ready to think about it just yet, put this section aside and come back to it later.

Getting Your House in Order

The most useful way to come to terms with your eventual death is to take positive steps to prepare for it. This means to "get your house in order" by attending to all the small and large details that are necessary. If you continue to avoid dealing with these details, you will create problems for yourself and for those who will become involved with your situation in a significant way. There are several components to getting your house in order:

- *Decide, and then convey to others your wishes about how and where you want to be during your last days and hours.* Do you want to be in a hospital or at home? When do you want procedures to prolong your life stopped? At what point do you want to let nature take its course when it is determined that death is inevitable? Who should be with you: only the few people who are nearest and dearest, or all the people you care about and want to see one last time?

- *Make a will.* Even if your estate is a small one, you may have definite preferences about who should have what. If you have a large estate, the tax implications of a proper will may be very significant.

- *Make arrangements, or at least plans, for your funeral.* Your grieving family would be very relieved not to have to decide what you would want and how much to spend. There are prepaid "future need" funeral plans available, and you can purchase burial space where and of the type you prefer.

- *Make a Durable Power of Attorney for Health Care* (see Chapter 11) and also one that will let someone manage your financial affairs. You should also discuss your wishes with your personal physician, even if he or she doesn't seem to be very interested. (Your physician may also have trouble facing the prospect of losing you.) Be sure that some kind of document or notation is included in your medical records that indicates your wishes in case you can't communicate them when the time comes.

- *Be sure that the persons you want to handle things after your death are aware of all that they need to know*—about your wishes, your plans and arrangements, and the location of necessary documents. You will need to talk to them, or at least prepare a detailed letter of instructions, and give it to someone who can be counted on to deliver it to the proper person when needed. This should be a person close enough to you to know when that time is at hand. You may not want your spouse or partner to have to take on these responsibilities, for example, but he or she may be the best person to keep your letter and to know when to give it to your designated agent. You can purchase at any well-stocked stationery store a preorganized kit in which you place a copy of your will, your Durable Power of Attorney, important papers, and information about your financial and personal affairs. The kit also contains forms that you fill out about bank and charge accounts, insurance policies, the location of important documents, your safe deposit box and where the key is kept, and so on. This is a handy, concise way of getting everything together that anyone might need to know about.

- *"Finish business" with the world around you.* Mend your relationships. Pay your debts, both financial and personal. Say what needs to be said to those who need to hear it. Do what needs to be done. Forgive yourself. Forgive others.

- *Talk about your feelings about your death.* Most family and close friends are reluctant to initiate such a conversation but appreciate it if you bring it up. You may find that there is much to say and to hear from your loved ones. If you find that they are unwilling to listen to you talk about your death and the feelings that you are perceiving, find someone who will be comfortable and empathic in listening to you. Your partner, family, and friends may be able to listen to you later on. Remember, those who love you will also go through the stages of grieving when they have to think about the prospect of losing you.

Dying

A large component in fear of death is the fear of the unknown. "What will it be like?" "Will it be painful?" "What will happen to me after I die?"

Most people who die of a disease are ready to die when the time comes. Painkillers and the disease process itself weaken body and mind, and the awareness of self diminishes without the realization that this is happening. Most people just "slip away," with the transition between the state of living and that of no longer living hardly identifiable. Reports from people who have been "brought back to life" after being in a state of "clinical death" indicate they experienced a sense of peacefulness and clarity and were not frightened.

However, a dying person may sometimes feel very lonely and abandoned. Regrettably, many people cannot deal with their own emotions when they are around a person they know to be dying and so deliberately avoid their company, or they may engage in superficial chit-chat, broken by long awkward silences. This is often puzzling and hurtful to the dying person, who needs companionship and solace from those they counted on.

You can help by telling your partner, family, and friends what you want and need from them—attention, entertainment, comfort, practical help, and so on. Again, when a person has something positive to do, they are more able to cope with their emotions. If you can engage your loved ones in specific activities, they can feel needed and can relate to you around the activity. This will give you something to talk about, to occupy time, or at least provide a definition of the situation for them and for you.

If you choose to die at home, a *hospice* can be very helpful. Hospice organizations provide both physical and emotional care to people who are dying, as well as for their families.

Suggested Reading

Carroll, David. *Living With Dying: A Loving Guide for Family and Close Friends.* New York: Paragon House, 1991.

Langone, John. *Death is a Noun: A Review of the End of Life.* Boston: Little, Brown, 1972.

Lewinsohn, Peter, with Ricardo Munoz, Mary Youngren, and Antoinette Zeiss. *Control Your Depression.* Englewood Cliffs, N.J.: Prentice Hall, 1987.

Martelli, Leonard J., Fran D. Peltz, William Messina, and Steven Petrow. *When Someone You Know Has AIDS: A Practical Guide.* New York: Crown, 1993.

Riley, Miles. *Set Your House in Order.* Garden City, N.J.: Doubleday, 1980.

Stedford, Averil. *Facing Death.* London: Wm. Heineman Medical Books, 1984.

Worden, J. William and William Proctor. *PDA—Personal Death Awareness.* Englewood Cliffs, N.J.: Prentice Hall, 1976.

16

Finding Resources

Amajor part of becoming a self-manager of your HIV/AIDS is knowing when you need help and how to find help. Seeking help to perform daily tasks, to assist with chores, or to help with other areas of your life does *not* mean that you have fallen victim to your illness. Instead, knowing where to go for help in specific areas of your life takes initiative, evaluation of your condition and your own capabilities. By becoming more aware of the symptoms you experience throughout the day, you can better predict the amount of energy and patience you will have to accomplish tasks. If you find that you come up short on energy, time, patience, or capability for some tasks, you can evaluate where help from other resources will save your own resources for those things most important to you.

The first resource you will probably go to for help is *family* or *close friends*. Some find it difficult, however, to ask for help from people they know. Finding the right words to ask for help is discussed in Chapter 10, "Communicating." Unfortunately, some people either do not have family or close friends to call on or cannot bring themselves to ask. If this is the case, you must look for other resources in your community. This chapter will show you how to search for resources and lists some of the most useful sources for the kind of help and information commonly needed by people with HIV/AIDS.

Getting Started—Finding Clues and Networking

Finding resources in your community is a little like a treasure hunt—creative thinking wins the game. Finding what you need may be as simple as looking in the telephone book and making a couple of phone calls. Other times, you will need to follow clues, including starting over when the clue leads to a dead end.

Where do you start? Suppose you find it difficult to prepare meals because prolonged standing is too tiring or painful. After some thought, you decide that you want to continue cooking for yourself rather than have someone else cook your meals. The next step, then, is to explore getting your kitchen altered so you can prepare meals from a seated position. Where can you find an architect or contractor who has knowledge and experience in kitchen alterations for people with physical limitations? Looking at the yellow pages and the classified section of the newspaper reveals pages of ads and listings for architects and contractors; some ads say they specialize in kitchens, while others don't mention any specialty. None mention anything about designing for physical limitations. A couple of phone calls to contractors listing kitchens as a specialty are unsuccessful in finding anyone experienced in kitchens for the physically limited.

Now what? You could call everyone listed until you find what you need. Not only would this be time consuming, but you may not feel comfortable about the contractor you find until you talk to someone else who knows this person's work. Here is where creative thought and networking enter the picture. Who else do you know that might have information of this kind? Maybe someone who works with physically disabled people would have ideas —an occupational or physical therapist, an orthopedic supply store, your city or county's human services department or commission, the nearest independent living center for the disabled, the community college disabled services office, or your local AIDS service organization. You may talk to someone who doesn't have the answer but says, "Gosh, Jack So-and-So just had his kitchen remodeled to accommodate his wheelchair. Maybe he can help you find someone." Jack's name is probably a great lead to follow. He may be able to give you not only the name of someone who does the work, but also some ideas about cost and other concerns before you go any further in the process. He's probably done much of the groundwork already and can save you time and trouble.

Suppose, however, that your search still isn't successful? Every community has people who are natural resources. These "naturals" seem to know everyone and know where everything is. They tend to be folks who have lived in the community a long time, and have been involved in it. They are natural problem solvers—the one people always seek out for advice. If you were to call this person, he or she would probably know the answer or set you on the right path to get the answer. The "natural" could be a friend, a business associate, the mail carrier, your physician, your pet's veterinarian, the checker at the corner grocery, the pharmacist, the bus or taxi driver, your child's school secretary, a realtor, the chamber of commerce receptionist, or the librarian. All you need do is think of this person as an information resource.

Resources for Resources

As in the two examples above, most searches for information begin with a single step and expand into a web of networking that will bring you into contact with unexpected resources.

The following list will give you many starting points for finding the resources you need:

- *The telephone book* is where most people start to look for community resources. Particularly if you need to hire someone to do something for you, the telephone book is full of people and organizations ready to help you.

- *Local AIDS information and referral services* will be listed in your telephone book. Look under AIDS Information and Referral, United Way Information and Referral, or "information and referral" in your county or city government listings. Once you have an information and referral telephone number, your searches will become much easier. These services maintain a huge file of referral addresses and telephone numbers for just about any help you might need. Even if they don't have the answer to your need, they will almost always be able to refer you to another agency that can speed you along in your search.

- *Voluntary agencies dedicated to your disease* are one of the most important resources you can find for either information or help. For people with HIV/AIDS, this means your local AIDS Foundation. Agencies of this type are funded by contributions from individuals and corporate sponsors and provide up-to-date information about your disease as well as support and direct services to people with AIDS. For a small membership fee, you can become a member of these organizations, which entitles you to receive regular bulletins by mail. You do not however, have to be a member to qualify for their services. They are here to serve you.

- *National HIV/AIDS organizations* maintain telephone hotlines to offer information about all kinds of resources, many of which may be available in your community.

- *HIV/AIDS resource guides* are often published by local HIV/AIDS organizations and provide information about services and resources available to people with HIV/AIDS. The listings are categorized by type—financial, medical, social, and mental health and support—and they are updated regularly.

- *Other community organizations, such as community centers and religious social service agencies,* also offer information and referral services as well as direct services. The latter may include classes, recreational opportunities, nutrition programs, legal and tax help, and social programs. There is probably a community center close to you. Your city government office or local librarian will know where they are, and the calendar section of your newspaper will usually have information about programs these organizations offer.

- *Religious groups* usually offer information and social services to those in need, either directly through the local church or synagogue or through the Council of Churches, Catholic Charities, or Jewish social service groups. To get help from religious organizations, start with your local church or synagogue; they will help you or refer you to someone who can help. You need not be a member of the religion or of its local organization to receive help.

- *Hospital and health care organizations* may also offer services. Many clinics caring for people with HIV/AIDS have access to excellent social workers and case managers who can give you much help. Call your local hospital, clinic, or health insurance plan and ask for their social service department. *Your doctor* will also be aware of the services available in the health care organizations he or she is affiliated with.

- *Libraries* are invaluable resources, particularly when you are looking for information about your disease. The library, and the *reference librarian* in particular, can serve as an information and referral service as well. Often the reference section of the library will have a gem of a book or pamphlet that will give you listings of the resources you are looking for. The reference librarian can probably take you right to it—and perhaps show you others as well. Even if you think you are good at library research, it's a good idea to ask the reference librarian if you have overlooked something. Reference librarians see volumes of material cross their desks and are knowledgeable about community resources.

- *University and college libraries* are also open to the public. By law, in fact, the regional *government documents* sections of these libraries must be open to the public at no charge. Government publications exist on just about any subject, and the health-related publications are particularly extensive. You can find information on everything from organic gardening to detailed nutritional recipes. The librarians are usually very helpful, and these publications are "your tax dollars at work."

- *Medical school libraries*, if you are fortunate enough to have one in your community, are another resource for information (although they are not a place to look for help with tasks). Naturally, you would expect to find a great deal of information about disease and treatment at a medical library, but unless you have some special knowledge about medicine, the information you find there can be intimidating and confusing. Use medical libraries with care.

- *Backs of books* are another great resource. Look for the reading lists (sometimes titled "Bibliography") and other resource lists at the back of books related to your disease. Sometimes this information is easy to miss because it is found just before or after the index. Backs of books are helpful for finding information as well as names and addresses of agencies and other organizations.

- *Local newspapers* are an excellent source of information. The health or science editor and the calendar of events editor can also be very knowledgeable about community resources. Gay community newspapers in particular contain a great deal of information. Two newspaper sections that can be most helpful in your search for resources are the *calendar of events section* and the *classified section*. Organizations advertise classes, lectures, and other events in both of these sections. In the classifieds, look under "Announcements," "Health," or any other heading that looks promising (you'll find an index of the headings used by your newspaper printed at the front of the classified section). Even if you are not interested in the particular events advertised, the contact telephone numbers may be good leads in your search for something else. Look in other logical places for news stories that might also be of interest, such as the pages around the calendar section or the health and fitness section (you might find an exercise program for people with your health problem there, for example).

- *The Internet* is an almost endless source of information about HIV/AIDS. Of course, you have to have access to a computer that is on the Internet (either by modem or directly linked), and you have to be comfortable using the computer. But if you can solve these problems, the Internet can be a way to look up treatment options, ask questions, find out about studies—all kinds of information. The great thing about the

Internet is that literally everything is there. The not-so-great thing about the Internet is that . . . literally everything is there. Anyone can put anything they want on the Internet. There's no one editing the material. The quality can really vary.

So how does one separate what's valid from what's not valid (or even crazy)? It can be hard to tell. On the World Wide Web, sites created by official organizations (like the CDC, or universities, or the major AIDS organizations) are reliable, and they generally have material that's in the mainstream of thought about AIDS. Information from news groups or "personal" web sites is often more interesting, but you may need to treat much of it skeptically. People may try to sell you things—look out for extravagant claims about new "cures." Discuss things you've heard about on the internet with others. If something sounds too good to be true, it probably is.

All of these resources are just first steps. Once you've started down any path, you'll find that with persistence and creativity, your information and support network will grow to give you many choices. You are not alone.

A Reference Guide of HIV/AIDS-Related Telephone Numbers

National Hotlines

If you need information, counseling, or referrals, these numbers will get you started. The National AIDS Hotline is accessible 24 hours a day in case your state hotline has closed for the evening and you need someone to talk to.

Centers for Disease Control and Prevention (CDC)

National AIDS Hotline .... *(800) 342-2437*

> Open 24 hours a day. Offers everything a state hotline does, including trained counselors. If you need referrals to local agencies or services, your state hotline number may have more up-to-date information.

National AIDS Clearinghouse .... *(800) 458-5231*

> Accesses all of the CDC's published information. You can get referrals to AIDS service organizations and services, order publications, get information about AIDS in the workplace, find out about the latest clinical trials, or use an automated service to get information via fax. You can also order a free catalogue of HIV/AIDS education and prevention materials.

HIV/AIDS Treatment Information Service .... *(800) 448-0440*

> Provides federally approved treatment guidelines for HIV and AIDS for health-care providers and people living with HIV infection.

HIV/AIDS Media Inquiries .... *(404) 639-3286*

Fax Information Service .... *(404) 332-4565*

National Institutes of Health

AIDS Clinical Trials Information Service .... *(800) TRIALS-A*

> Provides up-to-date information on clinical trials that evaluate experimental drugs and other therapies for adults and children at all stages of HIV infection.

Government trials at NIAID/NIH .... *(800) 243-7644*
Conducted in Maryland; all expenses covered.

National Institute of Allergy and Infectious Diseases (NIAID)
NIAID Division of AIDS .... (301) 496-0545
NIAID Press Office .... (301) 402-1663

Food and Drug Administration
Antiviral Agents Committee .... (800) 741-8138

Community Contacts
ACT UP (nationwide information) .... (215) 731-1844
AIDS Project/Los Angeles .... (213) 993-1600
AIDS National Interfaith Network .... (202) 546-0807
American Foundation for AIDS Research .... (202) 331-8600
American Institute of Teen AIDS Prevention .... (817) 237-0230
Gay and Lesbian Alliance Against Defamation .... (212) 807-1700
Gay Men's Health Crisis AIDS Hotline .... (212) 807-6655
Indian AIDS Hotline .... (800) 283-2437
National Association of People with AIDS .... (202) 898-0414
National Hemophilia AIDS Foundation .... (800) 424-2634
National Lesbian and Gay Health Association .... (202) 939-7880
National Minority AIDS Council .... (202) 483-6622
National Women's Health Network .... (202) 347-1140
People with AIDS Coalition Hotline .... (800) 828-3280
People with AIDS Health Group .... (212) 255-0520
Project Inform Treatment Hotline .... (800) 822-7422
San Francisco AIDS Foundation .... (415) 487-3000
Seattle Treatment Education Project .... (800) 869-7837
SIDA (Spanish Information Hotline) .... (800) 344-7432
Test Positive Aware Network (TPA) .... (312) 404-8726

State AIDS Hotlines

It is impossible to list all the AIDS service organizations that exist nation-wide. The following hotlines have up-to-date information and can refer you to an agency near you, whatever your needs may be.

State	Number	State	Number
Alabama	(800) 228-0469	Nebraska	(800) 782-2437
Alaska	(800) 478-2437	Nevada	(800) 842-2437
Arizona	(602) 265-3300	New Hampshire	(800) 752-2437
Arkansas	(800) 364-2437	New Jersey	(800) 624-2377
N. California	(800) 367-2437	New Mexico	(800) 545-2437
S. California	(800) 922-2437	New York	(800) 872-2777
Colorado	(800) 252-2437		(800) 541-2437
Connecticut	(800) 203-1234	North Carolina	(800) 342-2437
Delaware	(800) 422-0429	North Dakota	(800) 472-2180
Washington, DC	(202) 332-2437	Ohio	(800) 332-2437
Florida	(800) 352-2437	Oklahoma	(800) 535-2437
Georgia	(800) 551-2728	Oregon	(800) 777-2437
Hawaii	(800) 922-1313	Pennsylvania	(800) 662-6080
Idaho	(208) 345-2277	Puerto Rico	(809) 765-1010
Illinois	(800) 243-2437	Rhode Island	(800) 726-3010
Indiana	(800) 848-2437	South Carolina	(800) 322-2437
Iowa	(800) 445-2437	South Dakota	(800) 592-1861
Kansas	(800) 232-0040	Tennessee	(800) 525-2437
Kentucky	(800) 654-2437	Texas	(800) 299-2437
Louisiana	(800) 922-4379	Utah	(800) 366-2437
Maine	(800) 851-2437	Vermont	(800) 882-2437
Maryland	(800) 638-6252	Virgin Islands	(809) 773-2437
Massachusetts	(800) 235-2331	Virginia	(800) 533-4148
Michigan	(800) 872-2437	Washington	(800) 272-2437
Minnesota	(800) 248-2437	West Virginia	(800) 642-8244
Mississippi	(800) 826-2961	Wisconsin	(800) 334-2437
Missouri	(800) 533-2437	Wyoming	(800) 327-3577
Montana	(800) 233-6668		

AIDS-Related Publications

AIDS Treatment News .... *(800) 873-2812*
  Biweekly developments in research, experimental
  therapies, politics, and treatments

Being Alive .... *(213) 667-3262*
  Newsletter published by People with HIV/AIDS
  Coalition/LA

BETA .... *(800) 959-1059*
  San Francisco AIDS Foundation quarterly

Body Positive .... *(212) 566-7333*
  Nontechnical monthly magazine for people who
  are HIV-positive

Critical Path AIDS Project .... *(215) 545-2212*
  AIDS Library of Philadelphia monthly

*HIV/AIDS Resources: The National Directory
of Resources on HIV Infection/AIDS* .... *(800) 225-1860*
  Annual guide of nationwide services, education,
  prevention, hotlines, and medical facilities for
  HIV/AIDS

Media Resource Service .... *(800) 223-1730*

PI Perspectives .... *(800) 822-7422*
  Published by Project Inform with briefing papers
  issued between publications

PWA Newsline .... *(800) 828-3280*
  Newsletter published by People with HIV/AIDS
  Coalition/NY

Treatment Issues .... *(212) 337-3613*
  Monthly GMHC newsletter of experimental
  therapies. $30 donation requested; free to people
  with HIV/AIDS

Pharmaceutical Company Patient-Assistance Programs

The following is not a complete list of HIV/AIDS drugs, but a list of the more common drugs covered under indigent-patient programs. Each pharmaceutical company has different restrictions involving enrollment criteria, but most will not allow drug coverage in their health insurance policies, Medicare, Medicaid, or American Cancer Society grants.

Generic Name	Brand Name	Phone
Acyclovir	Zovirax	(800) 722-9294
Amitriptyline	Endep	(800) 285-4484
Atovaquone	Mepron	(800) 722-9294
Azithromycin	Zithromax	(212) 573-2820
AZT	Retrovir	(800) 722-9294
Bleomycin	Blenoxane	(800) 272-4878
Cefotaxime	Claforan	(800) 422-4779
Ceftriaxone	Rocephin	(800) 285-4484
Cefuroxime	Ceftin	(800) 452-9677
Cefuroxime	Kefurox	(800) 545-6962
Cimetidine	Tagamet	(800) 546-0420
Ciprofloxacin	Cipro	(800) 998-9180
Clarithromycin	Biaxin	(800) 688-9118
Clindamycin	Cleocin	(800) 242-7014
Clofazimine	Lamprene	(800) 257-3273
Clonazepam	Klonopin	(800) 285-4484
Clotrimazole	Lotrimin	(800) 656-9485
Clotrimazole	Mycelex	(800) 998-9180
Compazine	Prochlorperazine	(800) 546-0420
Cyclophosphamide	Cytoxan	(800) 272-4878
Cyclosporine	Sandimmune	(800) 447-6673
d4T	Zerit	(800) 736-0003
ddC	Hivid	(800) 285-4484
ddI	Videx	(800) 736-0003
Dexamethasone	Decadron	(800) 994-2111
Dronabinol	Marinol	(800) 274-8651
Doxycycline	Vibramycin	(800) 646-4455
Epoetin alfa	Epogen	(800) 272-9376
Epoetin alfa	Procrit	(800) 553-3851

(continued)

Generic Name	*Brand Name*	*Phone*
Ethambutol	Myambutol	(800) 533-2273
Erythromycin	A/T/S	(800) 422-4779
Famciclovir	Famvir	(800) 546-0420
Famotidine	Pepcid	(800) 994-2111
Fentanyl	Duragesic	(800) 544-2987
Fluconazole	Diflucan	(800) 869-9979
Flucytosine	Ancobon	(800) 285-4484
Fluocinonide	Lidex	(800) 822-8255
Foscarnet	Foscavir	(800) 488-3247
Ganciclovir	Cytovene	(800) 444-4200
G-CSF (Filgrastim)	Neupogen	(800) 272-9376
Gentamicin	Garamycin	(800) 656-9485
Granisetron	Kytril	(800) 866-6273
GM-CSF	Leukine	(800) 334-6273
GM-CSF	Prokine	(800) 656-9485
Human Growth Hormone	Nutropin	(800) 879-4747
Human Growth Hormone	Protropin	(800) 879-4747
Human Growth Hormone	Humatrope	(800) 545-6962
Hydrocortisone	Hydrocortone	(800) 994-2111
Hydrocortisone	Cortef	(800) 242-7014
Hydroxyzine	Atarax/Vistaril	(800) 646-4455
Immune Globulin	Gamimune	(800) 998-9180
Interferon Alpha-2	Roferon-A	(800) 443-6676
Interferon Alpha-2	Intron A	(800) 521-7157
Itraconazole	Sporanox	(800) 544-2987
Ketoconazole	Nizoral	(800) 544-2987
Liposomal doxorubicin	DaunoXome	(800) 247-3303
Loperamide	Imodium	(800) 544-2987
Loratadine	Claratin	(800) 656-9485
Megestrol acetate	Megace	(800) 736-0003
Methotrexate	Rheumatrex	(800) 533-2273
Methylprednisolone	Medrol	(800) 242-7014

(continued)

Generic Name	Brand Name	Phone
Mexiletine	Mexitil	(800) 556-8317
Morphine sulfate	Roxanol	(800) 274-8651
Nimodipine	Nimotop	(800) 998-9180
Nizatidine	Axil	(800) 545-6962
Nystatin	Mycostatin	(800) 272-4878
Octreotide acetate	Sandostatin	(800) 447-6673
Paclitaxel	Taxol	(800) 272-4878
Paromomycin	Humatin	(800) 755-0120
Pentamidine	NebuPent	(800) 366-6323
Pentoxifylline	Trental	(800) 366-6323
Phenytoin	Dilantin	(800) 755-0120
Prednisone	Deltasone	(800) 242-7014
Prednisone	Meticorten	(800) 656-9485
Prochlorperazine	Compazine	(215) 751-5722
Pyrazinamide	PYR500, PZA	(800) 533-2273
Pyrimethamine	Daraprim	(800) 722-9294
Pyrimethamine/Sulfadoxine	Fansidar	(800) 285-4484
Ranitidine	Zantac	(800) 452-9677
Rifabutin	Mycobutin	(800) 795-9759
Rifampin	Rimactane	(800) 257-3273
Scopolamine	Transderm-Scop	(800) 257-3273
Streptomycin	S. USP	(800) 646-4455
Sucralfate	Carafate	(800) 362-7466
Terfenadine	Seldane	(800) 362-7466
Testosterone	Testoderm	(415) 962-4243
TMP/SMX	Septra	(800) 722-9294
TMP/SMX	Bactrim	(800) 285-4844
Trimetrexate	NeuTrexin	(800) 887-2467
Valaciclovir	Valtrex	(800) 722-9294
Vinblastine	Velban	(800) 545-6962
Vincristine	Oncovin	(800) 545-6962
VP16 (Etoposide)	VePesid	(800) 272-4878

State Prescription-Drug Assistance Programs

State assistance can be an excellent source of benefits for people with HIV/AIDS. Don't assume that your income level is too high to be eligible for publicly funded programs. You can have a job, a car, a home, and *some* savings. Depending on the circumstances, a person may be able to receive free prescription drugs or financial assistance.

Call the number for your state to find out what's available. Many states no longer have a T-cell restriction simply because every person's treatment and prophylaxis regimen is unique, especially pregnant women and children with HIV/AIDS. You will need a prescription from a physician or an application showing your HIV status and your need for assistance. (If you have Medicaid or Medicare, chances are you will not qualify.) If you don't have a primary care physician or a case manager, the numbers on this page may help you get one and will also offer a number of other services.

Alabama	(334) 613-5364
Arkansas	(501) 376-6299
Arizona	(602) 230-5819
California	(916) 327-6781
Colorado	(800) 858-2437
Connecticut	(800) 233-2503
DC	(202) 347-8888
Delaware	(302) 995-8653
Florida	(904) 922-6675
Georgia	(404) 657-3129
Hawaii	(808) 732-0315
Idaho	(208) 334-6657
Illinois	(800) 825-3518
Indiana	(317) 920-3190 ext. 314
Iowa	(515) 242-5838
Kansas	(913) 296-8891
Kentucky	(502) 564-6539
Louisiana	(504) 568-5304
Massachusetts	(800) 228-2714

Maine	(207) 287-5060
Michigan	(517) 335-9333
Minnesota	(800) 657-3761
Mississippi	(601) 960-7723
Missouri	(314) 751-6439
Montana	(406) 444-4744
Nebraska	(402) 559-4673
Nevada	(702) 687-4800
New Hampshire	(800) 852-3345 ext. 4480
New Jersey	(609) 588-7038
New Mexico	(800) 545-2437
New York	(800) 872-2777
North Carolina	(919) 733-3091
North Dakota	(701) 328-2378
Ohio	(614) 466-6669
Oklahoma	(800) 285-2273
Oregon	(503) 731-4029
Pennsylvania	(800) 922-9384
Puerto Rico	Contact public health clinic
Rhode Island	(401) 464-2183
South Carolina	(800) 856-9954
South Dakota	(800) 592-1861
Tennessee	(615) 741-8903
Texas	(800) 255-1090
Utah	(801) 538-6197
Vermont	(800) 987-2839
Virginia	(804) 225-4844
Washington	(800) 272-2437
West Virginia	(304) 345-4673
Wisconsin	(608) 267-6875
Wyoming	(307) 777-5800

Services for Ethnic and Other Minority Groups

General

The Office of Minority Health .... *(800) 444-6472*
Leadership, advocacy, and information resources
for minority populations, including African-
Americans, Asian-Pacific Islanders, Latinos,
and Native Americans

The National Minority AIDS Council. .... *(800) 559-4145*
Advocacy for minority groups

If you are interested in HIV issues more specific to a particular ethnic group,
ask for a referral or call one of the following numbers:

African-Americans

American Red Cross, African-American
    HIV/AIDS Program .... (703) 206-7411
National Task Force on AIDS Prevention .... (415) 356-8100
Black, Gay, and Lesbian Leadership Forum .... (213) 964-7820
Howard University, National AIDS Minority
    Information and Education Program .... (202) 865-3720
National Black Women's Health Project .... (404) 758-9590

Asian-Pacific Islanders

Asian and Pacific Islander American Health Forum ...... (415) 541-0866
National Asian-Pacific American Families
    Against Substance Abuse .... (213) 278-0031
Organization of Chinese American Women .... (202) 638-0330
Association of Asian-Pacific
    Community Health Organizations .... (510) 272-9536

Hispanics

American Red Cross, Hispanic
    HIV/AIDS Program .... (703) 206-7602
National Coalition of Hispanic Health and
    Human Services Organizations .... (202) 387-5000

National Council of La Raza . . . . (202) 785-1670

National Puerto Rican Coalition . . . . (202) 223-3915

Native Americans

National Native American
 AIDS Prevention Center . . . . (510) 261-2505

American Indian Health Care Association . . . . (800) 473-1926

National Congress of American Indians . . . . (202) 466-7767

Hearing- and Speech-Impaired

The following numbers are text telephone (TTY/TDD) numbers. The asterisk (*) indicates a voice and TTY line; you may have to tap the space bar to let them know it is a TTY call.

CDC National AIDS Clearinghouse . . . . (800) 243-7012

AIDS Clinical Trial Information Service . . . . (800) 243-7012

HIV/AIDS Treatment Information Service . . . . (800) 243-7012

Business and Labor Respond to AIDS
 Resource Service . . . . (800) 243-7012

AIDS Information Line . . . . (800) 551-2728

AIDS Project Inc. . . . . *(800) 851-2437

Department of Medical Assistance Services . . . . (800) 343-0634

Disability Rights Center, Inc. . . . . (800) 834-1721

San Francisco AIDS Foundation . . . . (415) 864-6606

National Association of People with AIDS . . . . *(202) 898-0414

Women

Women Organized to Respond to Life-Threatening
 Diseases (WORLD) . . . . (510) 658-6930

Women's Information & Service Exchange . . . . (404) 817-3441

National Resource Center on Women and AIDS . . . . (202) 872-1770

National Women's Health Network . . . . (202) 347-1140

National Women's Health Resource Center . . . . (202) 293-6045

17

Helpful Hints

It seems that we all have too much to do and not enough time and energy to do it, even when we are well. When we are coping with the effects of HIV/AIDS, anything that makes our lives a little easier becomes doubly important.

Fortunately, creative people before us have invented many, many short-cuts that make the tasks of everyday living run more smoothly. This chapter offers many energy-saving ideas grouped into activities from waking to sleeping, cooking to gardening, and from getting around inside to going out. Use the suggestions that appeal to you—we hope these lists will also jog your own imagination and problem-solving abilities. Write us and let us know what other ideas *you* come up with.

Waking Up

Try some stretching and strengthening exercises while you are still in bed.

Get a clock radio and set it to awaken you with music rather than an alarm. Some can wake you with a prerecorded tape of your choice. Record the tape with your own pep rally.

Make half of your bed while you are are still in it. Pull the top sheet and blanket up on one side and smooth them out. Exit from the unmade side, which is then easy to finish.

Use a quilted comforter with matching pillowcases or pillow shams instead of a bedspread. They are easy to pull up, and carefully smoothing the sheets and blankets underneath is unnecessary since the thick quilting hides any irregularities in the surface.

Do some of your dressing sitting on the edge of your bed before you get up. Leave the clothes within reach of your bed the night before.

Bathing and Hygiene

If standing in a shower or sitting down in a tub are too demanding, get a bath stool. It is waterproof and goes right in the tub. You can sit while you bathe.

Replaces shower heads or bath faucets with a unit that incorporates a hand-held sprayer.

A long, absorbent cotton terry robe will eliminate the effort of drying with a towel.

An oxygen tube can be kept out of the way while bathing by passing it over the shower curtain rod.

"Soap on a rope" enables you to use soap with one hand and keeps it from falling.

A liquid soap dispenser may be easier to use than a bar of soap.

If excess humidity bothers you, leave the bathroom door open while you bathe.

A "shower caddy" keeps bathing supplies within easy reach.

Use nonskid safety strips or a rubber bath mat in the tub or shower.

Consider having grab bars installed in your tub or shower to minimize the risk of falling.

Get a long-handled sponge or brush.

Have a grab bar or safety frame installed next to the toilet. A free-standing towel rack next to the toilet can also help you when getting off the toilet.

Women who are troubled by occasional incontinence (loss of urine) find that small panty-liners or sanitary pads with adhesive backs help avoid potentially embarrassing situations.

Women who find tampons difficult to remove might try winding the tampon

Bathing and Hygiene (continued)

string around a pencil and gently pulling with both hands. Some brands have looped strings, making removal with either fingers or a pencil easier.

Women who use pads for feminine hygiene can keep the genital area clean by using a squeeze bottle of water kept by the toilet. These bottles can be found with a variety of spray nozzles.

Dressing and Grooming

Shop for clothes with dressing in mind. Look for easy-to-reach fasteners, front openings, and comfortable waistbands loose enough to be pulled up easily.

When shopping for clothes, take a tape measure with you that is already marked with your measurements. By measuring the garments, you may not have to try on so many before you buy.

Lower the rod in your closet or get a closet organizer to bring clothes within easier reach.

If you are bothered by extreme temperatures, you may find cotton under-clothing more comfortable than synthetic.

Avoid tight belts, bras, or girdles that restrict chest and abdominal expansion.

Buy front-opening bras or fasten back-opening bras in front, then turn them around.

When putting on pantyhose or a girdle, roll them down from top to bottom, then step in, pull them up onto your hips, and unroll.

Using dusting powder on the thighs makes pulling on pantyhose or a girdle easier.

Most women find that wearing slacks and socks is much easier than struggling into pantyhose.

It is safer and easier to pull underpants and trousers up when lying flat in bed if balance or mobility are problems. Graduate to a chair.

Use a bent coat hanger, reacher, or "dressing stick" to help with pulling up pants or retrieving clothes that are out of reach.

Put rings or loops on zipper pulls, or get a special zipper puller.

Avoid tight neck bands. Ties should be loose, or replaced with a bolo or loosely tied scarf or kerchief.

Suspenders may be more comfortable than a belt.

Avoid socks or stockings with elastic bands or garters that may bind the leg and restrict circulation.

Use a sock donner to put on socks and stockings.

Get a long-handled shoehorn.

Slip-on type shoes are easy and require no bending over to tie.

Lace-up shoes are easier to tie with zipper laces.

Pants or skirts with pockets allow women to carry money, driver's license, and so on in the pockets instead of carrying a large, heavy purse.

Talk to a hair stylist about a no-fuss style. Special haircuts and/or perms can eliminate the extra effort needed to style hair.

If you have respiratory problems, switch to nonaerosol toiletries. Use liquid or gel hair dressings and roll-on or solid deodorants.

Use toiletries that are unscented or hypoallergenic if you are bothered by perfume.

Getting Around

Lead with your strongest leg when going up stairs. Lead with your weaker leg when going down.

Remove all throw rugs—they can cause falls.

Doorways inside your home can be made wider by removing the doors, making them easier to get through with a wheelchair, walker, or other equipment.

Consider installing stair rails on both sides of the stairway to increase safety.

A small ramp can replace a couple of stairs at the entrance to your home or elsewhere.

Carry a folding "cane seat" with you when you go out. It gives you both

Getting Around (continued)

something to lean on and something to sit on when necessary.

Look for a walker that has a large basket in front and a small bench seat to sit on when you get tired.

Consider installing a mechanical lift chair on your stairs.

Place a chair or table near the top of stairs for you to sit or lean on when you reach the top.

To lift and carry: (1) lift or carry while exhaling through pursed lips; (2) rest, and inhale through nose; (3) continue this pattern of intermittent work and rest until you get the job done.

Doing Household Chores

Get a small utility cart—some fold; most have at least two shelves. As you move about doing your chores, use the cart to carry your supplies or things that need to be put away. If you live in a two-story house, keep a cart on each level.

Plan your chores so that you go in a circle, rather than back and forth.

Keep a set of cleaning supplies in each area in which they are needed to avoid carrying them around.

A magnet tied to a string can help pick up thumbtacks, hairpins, and so on. It will stick to your cart, refrigerator, or washing machine for quick availability.

Pickup tongs can retrieve things from hard-to-reach places. The tongs can be purchased from most medical supply houses.

To clean your bathtub, sit on a low stool next to the tub and use a long-handled sponge.

Consider a battery-powered scrubber for bathtub and sink.

Get a long-handled dustbin and a small broom for dry spills. Small brooms can be found in toy stores.

Foam floor mats can be placed where you may need to stand often, such as at the sink, ironing board, or telephone. They can reduce foot and ankle pain, as well as low back pain.

If lifting heavy detergent boxes is difficult, have someone pour the soap into a small container, or put a large container on the floor and use a scoop.

For some, a front-loading washer is easier to use than a top-loader.

Wash small items such as socks or underwear in laundry bags to avoid having to search for them in the washer or dryer.

Use gravity to get clothes out of the dryer or front-loading washer. Put a basket under the door and scoop the clothes into it with a reacher or stick.

Try old-fashioned push-on clothespins rather than pinch clothespins.

Use an adjustable-height ironing board so you can sit down while ironing. Attach a cord minder to keep the cord out of your way.

If fitted bed sheets are difficult to put on the bed, slit one corner and fasten with a tie.

Use a large, wide spatula or oven shovel to tuck in sheets.

A small, battery-powered hand vacuum is easy to use for spot cleanups and can be kept on your cart.

Use a vacuum cleaner with disposable bags and remove the bag with extreme care if you have respiratory problems.

If you have breathing problems, avoid sweeping and dusting. If you feel you must do it, wrap the working end of the broom or mop with a damp cloth.

A damp cloth is also good for dusting. If you don't want to use anything damp on wood surfaces, get a roll of crinkly paper towels and a bottle of lemon oil. Tear the towels in sections and fold in quarters, put four or five coin-sized dots of oil on each towel, and roll up tight. Store in a zip-lock bag or a jar. Use and discard.

If you must do a dusty job, wear a mask.

Have good ventilation and an adequate supply of fresh air at all times.

People with respiratory problems should observe the no-aerosol rule for cleaning products.

Avoid harmful substances that can vaporize, such as mothballs, solvents, and kerosene.

Put lockable casters on furniture you wish to move to clean around.

Cooking

Microwave ovens save time and energy.

Replace the twist ties on bread or other foods with clothespins.

Avoid lifting heavy pots of food along with the water they were cooked in. Place food in a basket to lower into the water for cooking, or get a spaghetti cooker with a perforated insert. You can lift the basket out to drain food. Someone else can drain the pot later, or you can ladle it out.

Ask family members not to close jars too tightly. A jar opener can be mounted under a counter top, or you can get a rubber disk to help you open jars.

Try to replace any heavy cast-iron or ceramic utensils with lightweight pots, bowls, and dishes.

Don't try to get everything done at once. Almost all jobs can be divided into sections. For instance, clean the top shelf of the refrigerator today and the bottom shelf tomorrow.

Plan your meals when you are neither hungry nor tired. Light, well-balanced meals are too important to leave to impulse.

A number of small meals is better than large ones. Better for a person with limited lung capacity to allow more room for lungs than for the stomach.

Use convenience food when desired, but remember that many packaged foods have high salt and sugar contents. Read the labels.

Keep plenty of water in the refrigerator. You can get containers to sit on your shelf that have spigots near the bottom so you won't have to lift the container to fill your drinking glass.

For many recipes, it's just as easy to cook double or triple quantities as small ones. Freeze the excess in meal-sized containers and enjoy some cook-free meals when you feel like a day off. In a microwave, they can be easily thawed and heated without drying out.

A slow-cooker or crockpot can make many meals easier to prepare, as can a pressure cooker.

Always use an exhaust fan when cooking, especially if you have respiratory problems.

A small, portable fan can help you overcome shortness of breath from exertion or cool you off in a warm kitchen or laundry room. Some are battery powered and can clip on a shelf or counter.

Use your cart when tidying up after a meal. For example, gather all the items that need to go into the refrigerator and then sit down with the cart and put them away all at once.

Put your most-used pots and pans back on the stove and leave them there. Instead of putting dishes and silverware away, reset the table for the next meal.

Try a cutting board with spikes sticking up that will hold meat firmly in place while you cut it. If needed, you will be able to carve meat with one hand.

Select appliances with levers or pushbuttons that are easy to operate.

Store canned goods so that the same items are lined up behind one another. Storing them upside down allows you to see the labels easier.

Get attractive cooking pots that double as serving pieces.

Disposable foil pie tins, loaf pans, and so on save cleanup effort.

Line pans with aluminum foil for easier cleanup.

Get pans with a nonstick surface for quicker cleanup.

Stabilize mixing bowls by placing them on a wet washcloth or by placing them in an open drawer at work height.

Put flour and sugar in conveniently located containers so you won't have to lift the heavy bags.

Oven mitts allow you to lift hot pans with both hands.

Use a bent coathanger or a dowel with a hook on the end to pull out hot oven racks.

Attach a spray hose at the kitchen sink and fill pots with water while they sit on the countertop or stove.

A pizza wheel can cut more than pizza easily.

A small food processor can make short work of grating, chopping, or slicing.

Remembering Medications

A pillbox with a separate compartment for each day of the week is useful. You can make a homemade pillbox out of an egg carton or you can buy one ready-made at your pharmacy.

Some electronic pillboxes can be programmed to beep you when it's time to take your medication.

Take-out food places often have little, one-ounce plastic containers for salad dressing and ketchup that can be labeled and used for each pill-taking occasion during the day.

Associate your medication taking with a normal daily habit, such as brushing your teeth or watching the news. Put your pills next to the things you use for that activity (making sure your medications are out of the reach of children).

Whenever you get a prescription filled, figure out how long it will last and mark the time to reorder on a calendar. This reminder may save you from running out in the middle of the night or on a weekend or holiday.

Other Health Issues

Using a computer with access to the Internet is undoubtedly the best way to get information of all kinds about HIV/AIDS and its treatments.

To monitor your peripheral vision, use a regular newspaper and the Self-Test for Peripheral Vision, found in the Appendix. To monitor your central vision, use the Amsler Grid and the Self-Test for Central Vision, both also in the Appendix.

Buy a thermometer. You can't always tell whether you have a fever just by how you feel, and your temperature may not be high when you get to the doctor's office. Digital thermometers that are easy to read are widely available.

Shopping

Find grocery stores and pharmacies that deliver.

If you are shopping with an oxygen carrier, find a shopping cart on your way in and put the oxygen in it while you shop.

Some supermarket chains are now offering motorized, riding shopping carts.

When you are grocery shopping, have all the perishables packed in a separate bag. When you get home, put them away and leave the rest for later.

Community service clubs and churches will sometimes offer shopping services for people with disabilities. Volunteers will shop for you.

Mail-order catalogs offer just about everything you would want and are fun to look through, too. You need only be able to plan ahead a little.

If you have a home computer with access to the internet, you can do a lot of shopping by computer.

Going Out

Before going out, prepare for your homecoming. Lay out your comfortable clothes and slippers, leave a drink in a handy thermos, set out whatever utensils you will need for your evening meal, and even turn down your bed. Homecoming can then be a real relief.

Find out where you can get a daily air quality report for your area and use it when making your plans for the day.

Ask your doctor about getting a handicapped parking permit.

If you will have to sit in the car for a long period of time, make up a kit of helpful things such as a pad and pencil, paperback book, tissues, and so on. A coffee can with a snap-on plastic lid can be an emergency urinal.

If you worry about being away from a phone in an emergency situation, consider a CB radio or car phone. The expense may be worth it to get out and about without extra anxiety.

Get assertive about exposure to other people's tobacco smoke. You have a right to breathe smoke-free air. Ask smokers near you to stop.

If you must fill the gas tank, get upwind so you don't inhale the fumes.

Attach a loop to the inside door handle of your car to make it easier to pull closed.

Wide-angle rear-view mirrors allow for increased visibility without straining your neck.

Going Out (continued)

A back support device (such as Sacro Ease) can make a car seat much more comfortable.

When shopping for a new car, look for easy-to-open doors and easy-to-adjust seats.

Wash your hands well when you get home. Colds and other diseases are often spread by touch as well as through the air.

Gardening

Find lightweight, easy-to-handle tools. Many tools now come in lighter, durable plastic.

Use a folding stool or one with wheels. There are wheeled stools especially for gardening, with a tool storage area under the seat.

Many tools can be purchased with a long handle, or you can have a short handle replaced with a long one.

A riding mower, preferably with a self-starter, can be a real morale booster.

Enjoying Recreation and Leisure

Get to know your neighbors. Think of a signal, such as a pulled-down shade at night, to let them know you are OK.

Start a buddy phone system. Regular calls to and from friends are good for you, and these contacts will be able to aid in case of an emergency.

Somewhere near you, there is someone who needs your friendship and help, too. Look for these opportunities.

Home computers are getting more and more reasonable to own. Many games, including card and board games we all grew up with, are now available for home computers. You can have your own "Wheel of Fortune" game, with music and color graphics, right at home.

You can play board games long distance by mail or over the phone.

If you like to play cards, try a card holder.

Learn to use your computer or take art classes in an adult education class in your community. Your mind needs exercise, too, and you can meet interesting people in class.

Many adult education classes are offered through television or correspondence.

If you find your previous hobbies too demanding, try scaling them down for the time being. Start a container garden or try bonsai or orchids rather than a full-sized garden, for example.

If you like to paint, consider watercolors. They are lightweight and odorless and dry quickly.

An embroidery frame and stand will allow you to do needlework without having to use your hands to stabilize the piece you are working on.

Self-threading needles are available at yardage stores and through catalogs.

Traveling

Ask your doctor about your tolerance to altitude before you travel. Be aware of the altitudes of your destination, as well as altitudes while traveling to your destination.

You can arrange in advance with airlines for a wheelchair, special boarding and seating, or special meals. Be sure to call at least 24 hours in advance of your flight.

Travel light. Get suitcases with wheels or get a rolling luggage rack.

Ask your local disability access community group if there is a travel agent in your area who specializes in travel arrangements for people with physical limitations.

Getting Sleep

Go to bed in stages so that you arrive there relaxed, not worn out. Put on your nightclothes and then relax by reading or watching TV for a little while.

Have everything you need handy near your bed, such as a telephone and light. Have emergency numbers attached to the phone, or use a phone with

Getting Sleep (continued)

an auto-dial feature. A clock radio with earphones, a glass of water, and a urinal are also nice to have handy.

A night light will help to prevent falls and keep you from becoming disoriented in the dark.

Bedtime is often a good time to do some gentle muscle relaxation exercises.

Keeping Warm

Heating pads come in a variety of shapes and sizes to fit just about any part of your body.

Soak stiff, sore hands or feet in warm water.

Thermoelastic gloves are good for warming and are available in some pharmacies. Thermoelastic products are also available for knees and elbows.

Electric blankets and electric mattress pads are lightweight and warm.

Sleeping inside a sleeping bag placed under a blanket will help to keep you warm.

Consider long underwear. It comes in many colors and styles.

Preheat your bathroom before your bath or shower in the morning with a small space heater or heat lamp.

A large shawl is great for the occasional shivers, and much easier to put on and take off than a sweater.

Avoid really frigid temperatures if you have respiratory problems. Cold air can cause bronchospasms.

Appendix:
Self-Tests for Vision

You can do a self-test of your peripheral vision quite easily, using a common newspaper. If you use eyeglasses to read, be sure to wear them while you check your peripheral vision.

To test your peripheral vision, simply follow these instructions:

1. Open up a page of your newspaper and hold it out in front of you. The page should have mostly type on it, with few or no pictures.

2. Closing one eye, focus on any word at or near the middle of the page. Be sure to hold the page close enough so that printed words completely fill your field of vision (that is, so that print is all you can see).

3. Without moving your eye, notice if any area of the page seems darkened, blurred, or is missing. If you notice that any part of the page is out of focus, darkened, or missing entirely (even a small area), you should call your doctor right away!

4. Repeat this test for the other eye, following the same instructions. Be sure to test both eyes!

Self-Test for Central Vision Using the Amsler Grid

The image that appears on the next page is a version of the Amsler Grid. It can be used to regularly check your central vision for damage from cytomegalovirus (CMV) infection. You can do this test using the image as it appears in this book, or you can photocopy the image and use that to do the test. The grid image should appear approximately 5″ × 5″ square. If you wear glasses for reading, be sure to wear them while you check your central vision.

To test your central vision, simply follow these instructions:

1. Place the Amsler Grid image at a comfortable reading distance, about two feet away and with the image facing you squarely. The grid pattern should be clear and in focus.

2. Covering one eye with your hand, look directly at the dark square in the center of the grid. While looking only at this center square, look to see if the grid pattern immediately adjacent to the central dark square appears straight and even, like a piece of graph paper. If any of the lines appear distorted, blurred, discolored, or totally absent, you need to call your doctor right away!

3. Repeat the test for the other eye, following the same instructions above. Make sure you test both eyes, since CMV retinitis typically strikes only one eye at a time.

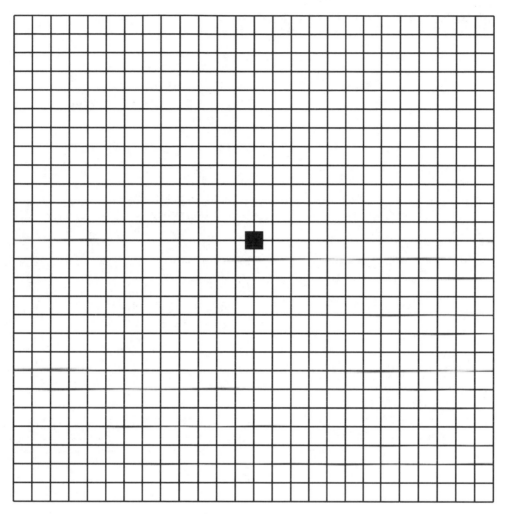

The Amsler Grid

Index